AF289855

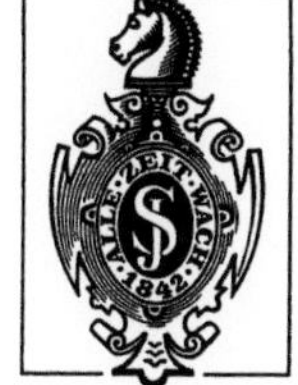

G. P. Marzoli   S. Vesentini

# Warren's Operation

With the cooperation of F. Frasson, C. Fugazzola
G. Mangiante, R. Maso

Foreword by A. Dagradi

With 46 Figures

Springer-Verlag
Berlin  Heidelberg  New York 1982

Professor Gian Pietro Marzoli*
Dr. Sergio Vesentini*
Dr. Franco Frasson**
Dr. Carlo Fugazzola**
Dr. Gerardo Mangiante*
Dr. Renzo Maso**

 * Clinica Chirurgica, Università Padova, Sede in Verona,
   Policlinico Borgo Roma, I-37100 Verona
** Istituto di Radiologia, Università Padova, Sede in Verona,
   Policlinico Borgo Roma, I-37100 Verona

ISBN-13:978-3-642-68110-3     e-ISBN-13:978-3-642-68108-0
DOI: 10.1007/978-3-642-68108-0

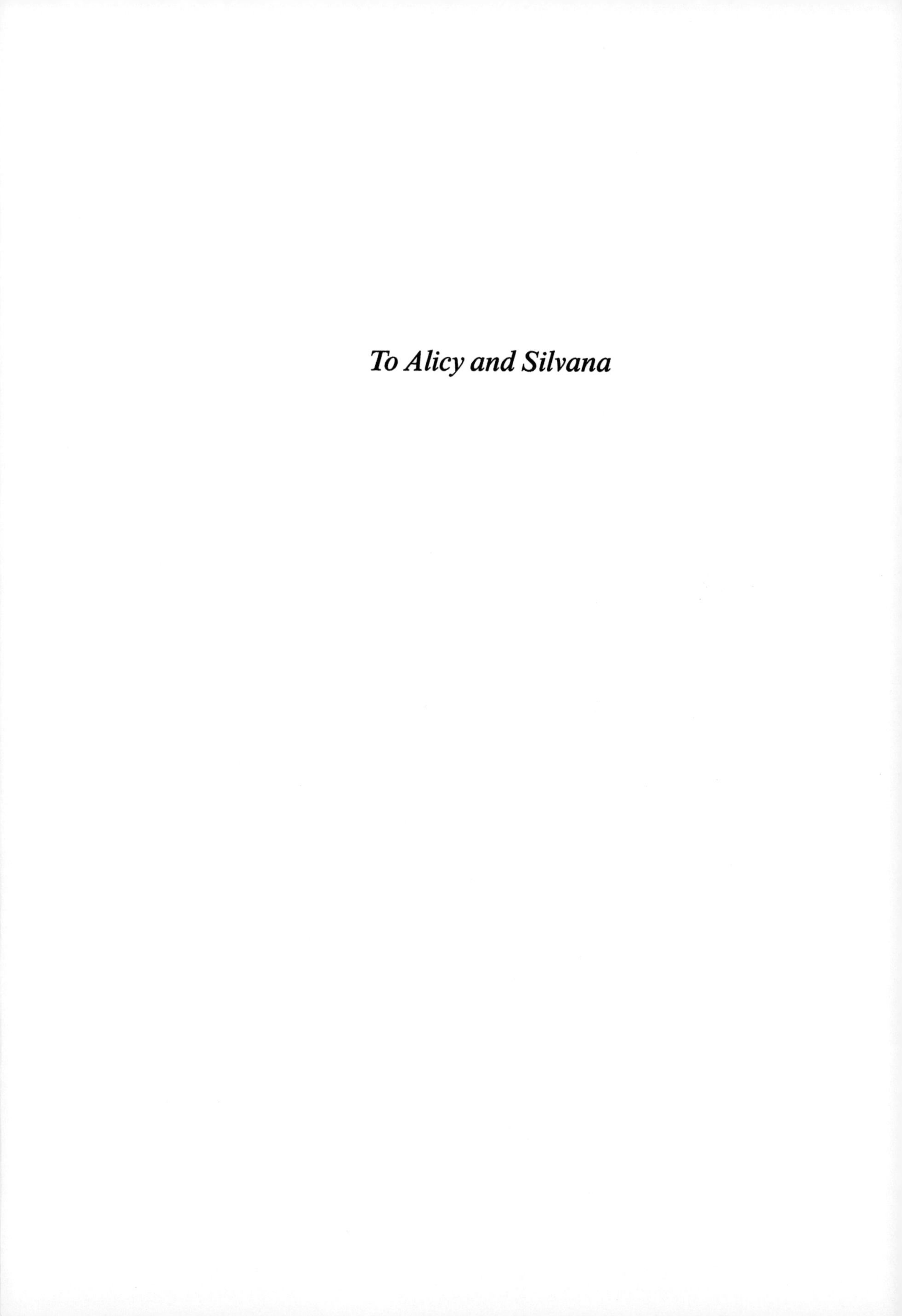

*To Alicy and Silvana*

# Foreword

I have particular pleasure in introducing this publication by
Gian Pietro Marzoli and Sergio Vesentini. Years ago they
enthusiastically accepted my suggestion that they should
take specific interest in the clinical and surgical problem of
portal hypertension, and assess the proposals of surgical experience with regard to this debated physiopathological
picture. These thanks are all the more real because in this
way the school's attention remained fixed on a subject that
had already attracted it profoundly from the start – with
Giovanni Castiglioni and Vittorio Pettinari as heads of the
school – and then threatened to die away into general con-
formism. In Italy "precariousness" is easily extended to the
concept of school continuity.

In Warren's proposal (1967) of "distal splenorenal anastomosis with disconnection of the spleno-oesophageal from
the mesenteric district", I felt there was an intelligent attempt to solve all the basic problems, albeit in different
ways. An attempt, that is to say, at alleviating the gastro-
oesophageal circulation, thus avoiding haemorrhage, and
at ensuring that the liver would maintain the circulatory efficiency with which it was still endowed. The spleen was retained, but there was reason to think that, by reducing blood
stasis within its ambit, it would be possible to manage or
alleviate any hypersplenism: not an absurd hypothesis if the
Americans had sometimes noted in their material functional and even anatomical reversion of the splenopathy after a
simple portacaval shunt. This vascular operation of Warren's was not the easiest from the technical standpoint, and
perhaps not even the most strikingly effective in cleansing
the oesophageal circulation; it might even be superfluous in
some cases (e. g. if the cirrhotic liver was now excluded from

portal transit), but in no case would it be harmful. In particular, it would evade the danger of encephalopathy.

Reasons could be found, if they were sought hard enough, for doubts about retention of the spleen in those patients in whom the extent of the hypersplenic damage insistently called to mind Banti's hypothesis. But I have already said that some advantage could be expected even in this direction, and it would be interesting to investigate the potential reversibility of these splenopathies as well. In line with these ideas, I asked my collaborators to make a clinical trial on Warren's operation, at first through a cautious approach to selected cases chosen on grounds of favourable physiopathological prospects and surgical technique, with the possibility of extension, according to confidence, and the immediate results.

I feel that they have reasonably, conscientiously, and ably progressed along this line.

That it would be useful to obtain practical assessment of Warren's conceptual approach from surgeons who, not being involved in its formulation, could ensure sufficient mental detachment from the method as to estimate the real extent of its effects, is a logic of clinical experimentation. In the surgeon's uneven path towards the ideal solution of the problem of "haemorrhagenic portal hypertension" probably the subsequent paper did not constitute a milestone, nor does the contribution I am introducing here seek to be such.

I feel that to gallop down a long, winding and treacherous road abounding in more or less attractive byways, in the blind faith of falling, by chance, on the next milestone showing that the road taken was the right one, is a source of blazing disappointments. Especially as it is very doubtful whether the milestone glimpsed from afar, or over which one stumbles accidentally, is really the right one. This milestone indeed may not yet have been placed and will only be placed with the combined effort of everybody.

Adamo Dagradi

# Preface

The purpose of this paper is not to hazard a judgment, which would certainly be premature, but to give an up-to-date balance sheet of the operation proposed by Warren, Zeppa, and Fomon in 1967. Warren's lucid and fascinating approach when putting forward the proposal for an operation (it is in fact an operation including a splenorenal shunt), aimed at avoiding the clinical consequences of a sudden and severe hepatic haemodynamic repercussion and directed to obtaining optimal prophylaxis against haemorrhagic relapse through selective drainage of the oesophago-gastro-splenic venous area alone, induced us to perform this operation in a group of portal hypertensive cirrhotic patients bleeding from varices.

Since Warren's approach to the operation is based mainly on haemodynamic considerations, we felt justified in not contenting ourselves with a mere recording of the clinical results. We have sought to make a haemodynamic check, mainly based on pre- and postoperative abdominal angiography (in some cases with long-term repetition), in order to record the behaviour of the portal circulation and the selectivity of the operation.

These pages are strictly linked to the subject "Warren's Operation"; deliberately, no account is taken of all the many problems of surgical treatment of portal hypertension in a wide sense. Space is given not only to the functional results, but also to the items of literature that specifically deal with the title subject.

We wish to express our gratitude to Prof. A. Dagradi, who set us on our way in this surgery.

Preface

Our thanks also go to Dr. Heinz Götze for taking up our proposal and assisting us in the publication of our paper.


*Acknowledgement*
We thank Dr. Gianfranco Briani and radiological technicians Marino Marini, Adriano Tommelleri and Claudio Merigo for their co-operation.


Verona, November 1981         G. P. Marzoli      S. Vesentini

# Contents

Contents

# 1. Introduction

Although the number of operations performed throughout the world for portal hypertension is put at over 100 000 [4] – and this is probably an underestimate – and although an enormous volume of work and experience has been accumulated on the subject, the problem of the ideal treatment of bleeding oesophageal varices due to portal hypertension still seems far from universally accepted solutions. This is demonstrated by the new operations continually proposed and the old operations proposed again with modifications [16, 41, 47, 48, 61].

In the western world, portal hypertension is mainly secondary to intrahepatic block induced by cirrhosis, generally of alcoholic and posthepatitic origin. It is with reference to this type of pathology that surgical treatment takes on highly complicated aspects centred on the trend of cirrhotic liver disease towards spontaneous evolution. This spontaneous trend is moreover not easy to quantify in relation to two other fundamental variables: the course of portal-systemic encephalopathy and the effect that all the operations have on hepatic portal perfusion.

The three variables and their interrelationships fully explain the difficulty of finding a solution of the clinical and therapeutic problems linked to portal hypertension.

All the operations adopted in the past and/or now in use – in addition to having a solely symptomatic significance – lack one or more of the following requisites, which may be considered ideal:
- No operative mortality
- Long-term survival unaffected
- Absolute prophylactic effectiveness
- Absence of repercussions on the basic liver disease
- No change in the haemodynamic status quo
- Absence of tendency to encephalopathic evolution

While it may have reached acceptable results as far as prophylactic effectiveness against haemorrhagic relapse, traditional portal hypertension surgery – based mainly on nonselective truncal and radicular shunt operations – leaves a good deal to be desired on other points, especially the considerable re-

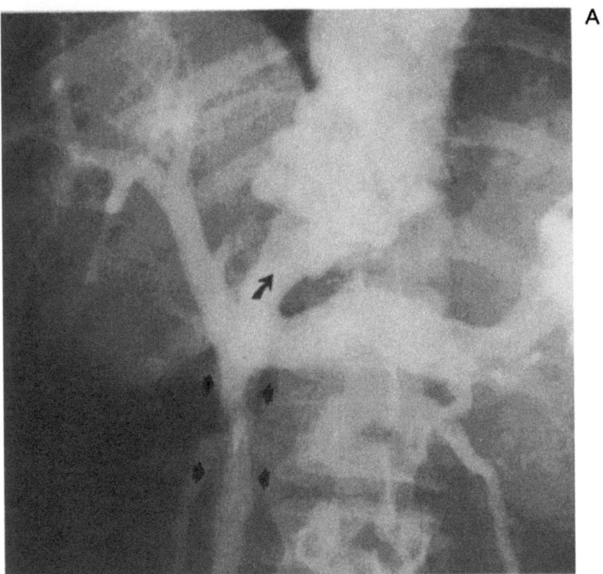

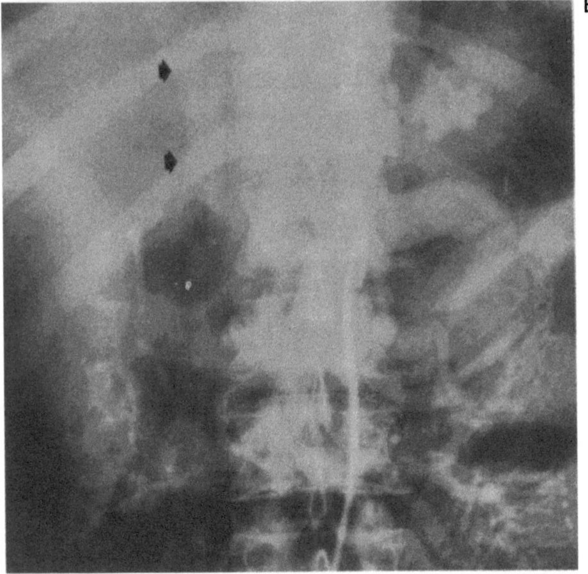

**Fig. 1 A, B.** Central splenorenal shunt with splenectomy.
**A** Pre-operative splenoportography. Splenic vein very dilated; retrograde filling of left gastric vein *(arrow)*, which feeds large oesophago-gastric varices, and of superior mesenteric vein *(arrows)*. Hepatopetal portal vein flow.
**B** Postoperative superior mesenteric angiography: venous fase. Patent anastomosis: distal tract of splenic vein, left renal vein and inferior vena cava *(arrows)* are clearly opacified. Oesophago-gastric varices are still evident, but noticeably reduced in size. The portal vein is not opacified in relation to the hepatofugal direction of blood flow

duction in portal hepatic perfusion with onset and/or aggravation of portal-systemic encephalopathy and the postulated negative effect on evolution of the cirrhotic liver disease [89].

Warren's operation [89] owes its proposal to observations (made during the 1960s) with regard to the development of ascites after terminolateral portacaval shunt and to investigations on the behaviour of portal hepatic perfusion after traditional shunt operations [95]. The large and immediate reduction found in portal hepatic perfusion after a considerable percentage of non-selective operations (Fig. 1) appeared to be responsible for hepatocellular hypoxic distress (the part played by compensatory hypertrophy of the hepatic artery is difficult to assess [10, 94]) –, as well as aggravation of the portal-systemic encephalopathy and depletion of the principles of enteric origin that are presumed to govern hepatic trophism and regeneration [72, 80].

These observations also led to the interpretation of a phenomenon widely observed in clinical practice: the great variability of individual response to portal-systemic shunts in terms of onset and aggravation of hepatic insufficiency. With onset of hepatic insufficiency and encephalopathy, the sudden and considerable shunt of the portal flow is tolerated less the more abundant the pre-operative hepatic portal perfusion. The proposal was therefore put forward

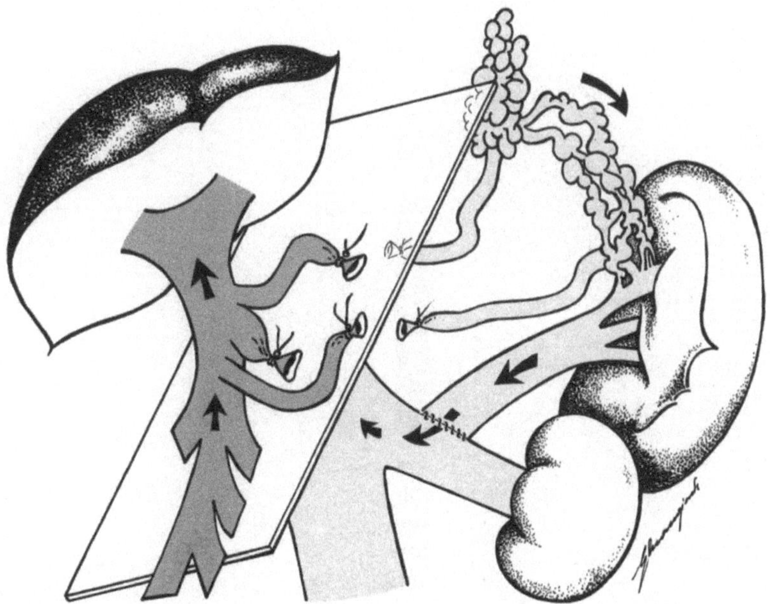

**Fig. 2.** Diagram of Warren's operation. The lighter part represents the low pressure zone drained by the shunt. The darker part represents the zone with unchanged portal pressure in maintenance of hepatic perfusion

that a pre-operative haemodynamic assessment should be made in order to identify patients at high haemodynamic risk who – since they possess good portal perfusion – are exposed to greater morbidity. However, the effectiveness of conventional angiographic observations in assessing the portal flow volume is sometimes disputed [9, 19, 22, 23, 54, 59, 72, 75, 76, 78].

An operation was devised on the basis of these physiopathological considerations, consisting mainly in a terminolateral splenorenal shunt and a gastro-oesophageal disconnection, with the following aims:

1. Selective drainage of the oesophagogastric varices through a distal splenorenal anastomosis
2. Preservation of portal perfusion by disconnection (Fig. 2) of the mesentericoportal bed from the hepatofugal flows to the varices (section of the right gastro-epiploic vein and right and left gastric veins), and
3. Separation of the enteric circulation into two parts: an oesophago-gastro splenic low pressure tract, drained into the systemic venous circulation through the splenorenal anastomosis, and a mesentericoportahepatic tract deprived of the splenic afflux, but also of the hepatofugal ducts to the varices.

# 2. Preliminary Investigations

Overall assessment of portal hypertensive patients who have certainly bled from oesophageal varices at least once, and hence are candidates for surgery, involves a series of investigations directed both to ascertaining the presence of a surgical indication (or the absence of contraindications) and selection of the method of operation.

*Taking for granted* the endoscopic diagnosis of bleeding from oesophageal varices, which is fundamental for avoidance of prophylactic operations, the subsequent steps are directed to:
1. Histological definition of the hepatic disease
2. Clinical and biochemical assessment of the hepatic functional reserve
3. Ascertainment of the existence and degree of encephalopathy
4. Morphological and functional (haemodynamic) study of the enteroportahepatic circulation [88].

## Histological Definition

Diagnosis of liver disease is essentially histological, on the basis of percutaneous or laparoscopic biopsy. The histological result is important both in clarifying the aetiology of the cirrhosis and in identifying morphofunctional data that can assist in the formulation of any contra-indications to the operation. These include, for example, the case of chronic hepatitis with considerable signs of activity, the existence of acute hyaline necrosis and the presence of Mallory-Weiss bodies, all conditions capable of endangering the operation.

## Clinical and Biochemical Assessment

The overall clinical assessment is based on objective data and biochemical data concerning general conditions, presence of ascites, presence of any other associated pathology, and hepatocellular efficiency as shown by the common hepatic function indices. (In particular, the maximal rate of urea synthesis

(MRUS) is to be recommended, although technically complex to determine [26].) The data thus collected can be used for a first evaluation of the operating risk (and hence of any contra-indications) according to Child's classification. It should, however, be remembered that patients do not always fit exactly into one of the three classes, due to discrepancies in respect of one or more indices [32].


## Ascertainment of Encephalopathy

An important factor in pre-operative assessment of patients consists in ascertainment of current portal-systemic encephalopathy [15, 55]. Recognition and evaluation of the encephalopathy are important from a number of standpoints, not least that of supplying a reference point in respect of the postoperative evolution of the encephalopathy. The diagnostic aspects of encephalopathy are complex, and it can probably be asserted that, provided sufficiently sophisticated procedures are used for its assessment, no cirrhotic is completely immune from it. However, a reasonable compromise between precision and practicality can be reached by adopting a routine diagnostic schedule including at least one EEG, ammonaemia, neuromuscular objective examination, and one of the numerous available psychometric tests [15].


## Functional Study of the Enteroportahepatic Circulation

Warren's operation imperatively demands a haemodynamic assessment as a fundamental factor in selection of the method of operation.

In current clinical practice such haemodynamic evaluation makes use of the following techniques:
1. Abdominal angiography with a study of the arterial and venous phases
2. Suprahepatic phlebography-manometry
3. Left renal phlebography
These examinations as a whole are defined as the "liver package" [59].


**a) Abdominal angiography,** performed by transfemoral route, involves injection of the contrast medium into the coeliac trunk, and selectively into the hepatic artery and splenic artery; study of the arterial and venous phases; selective injection of the superior mesenteric artery; and a further study of the arterial and venous phases, possibly aided in the last case by the administration of drugs [22]. The usable angiographic information has both morphological and functional significance.

The following parameters are assessed and recorded:
    Calibre and course of the hepatic and splenic arteries
    Volume of liver and intraparenchymal distribution of the arterial vessels
    Volume of spleen
    Endoluminal morphology of the splenoportal axis
    Calibre and direction of the portal vein
    Splenoportal axis ratios
    Portal flow volume and direction
    Existence of hepatofugal pathways
    Presence of ascites
    Associated hepatic pathology (tumours)

**b) Hepatic phlebography** is still a useful means of investigation, especially in regard to the aspects of manometric measurement of the occluding pressure (WHVP), which faithfully reflects the pressure conditions existing in the portal system [40, 72]. Hepatic injection of contrast medium is sometimes considered useful for visualization of the portal branches and hence an indication of the hepatofugal volume of portal perfusion [37, 59].

**c) Left renal phlebography** is an investigation to be carried out at the same time as suprahepatic phlebomanometry. With selective catheterization, not only the morphology and ratios of the left renal vein but also any pathological flow and pressure conditions can be recognised [59, 79].

Extremely valuable haemodynamic and morphological information can also be supplied by investigations such as splenoportography [1] with splenic manometry, and portography with manometry by umbilical route or transhepatic percutaneous route [72, 75, 78, 93]. The pressure readings obtained in this way may be considered to replace those given by suprahepatic phlebography, while the morphological aspects and those pertaining to demonstration of hepatofugal circulations are to be considered as a supplement to the data supplied by abdominal angiography.

Other haemodynamic informations are obtainable through scintiscanning techniques or dye-dilution tests [72]. These investigations can again be considered as a supplement to angiography. The fact that they are bloodless and non-invasive favours their use in assessment of postoperative hepatic portal perfusion [3], although the considerable criticisms on their validity should not be forgotten.

# 3. Indications – Contra-indications

Warren's operation can be considered the operation of first choice in the prevention of haemorrhagic relapses due to oesophageal varices in portal hypertensive patients. The operation is thus indicated in patients whose age and general conditions are compatible with a major operation, who have certainly bled from oesophageal varices at least once, and in whom the existence of portal perfusion can be demonstrated prior to operation.

The absolute contra-indication consists in intractable ascites, whereas failure to demonstrate portal perfusion constitutes a relative contra-indication, both because of the doubt about the validity of the observation and because of the theoretical indifference of such patients to any portal-systemic shunt. Other general contra-indicating factors consist in previous operations on stomach or pancreas, and previous episodes of acute or chronic pancreatitis; all these conditions are, in fact, capable of making the technical performance of the operation impossible (Fig. 3).

The points briefly enunciated above deserve some more detailed comments.

**Emergency**

Performance of Warren's operation in emergency conditions is not in itself contra-indicated, particularly if there has been an opportunity to carry out the appropriate angiographic investigations; the operation is in fact also performed in emergency conditions. A basic hindrance to emergency performance of Warren's operation consists in the technical difficulties it may offer, sometimes with very protracted operating times and hence harmful consequences on operative mortality [6]. Absence of information on permeability and the anatomical relations between the splenic vein and the left renal vein may lead to tardy intra-operative recognition that the shunt cannot be performed, with a further considerable time loss.

The fact remains that an adequate interval between the bleeding episode and surgical operation, during which medical treatment is given, leads to maxi-

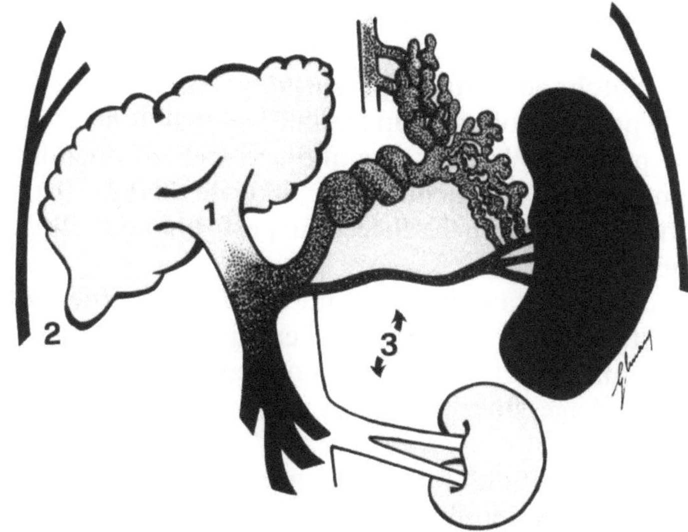

**Fig. 3.** Contra-indications to Warren's operation. *1*, reduced or absent portal hepatic pressure; *2*, intractable ascites; *3*, anatomical incompatibility

mal recovery of the hepatic function [91] and is therefore capable of ensuring reduced operative mortality as compared with emergency.

In our clinic, distal S-R shunts have not been performed in emergency conditions. In case of failure of the mechanical tamponing and transhepatoportal embolisation we perform a laterolateral portacaval shunt.


## Pathology

While the fundamental aetiological factor of portal hypertension in the western countries consists in alcoholic and posthepatitic hepatic cirrhosis, in the world as a whole the most frequent determining cause consists in intrahepatic blocks due to schistosomiasis [47]. In such cases Warren's operation is undoubtedly the ideal treatment [48].

In portal thrombosis, with cavernomatous transformation and partial recovery of portal perfusion, the condition may be considered "ideal" for Warren's operation, since the need is particularly felt to preserve as much as possible of the portal perfusion of an otherwise healthy liver [29, 47]. Complete portal thrombosis nullifies the physiopathological premises underlying selective operations.

## Age and General Conditions

In childhood portal hypertensions – nearly always due to prehepatic block – the principle of operating as late as possible still holds [47]. Moreover, in order to perform Warren's operation, vessels of adequate diameter are necessary, and hence it is difficult to carry it out at this age. In the literature there are nonetheless reports on the successful performance of this shunt in children [7, 45, 68, 86].

In adults, no limit beyond which not to operate can be fixed a priori. The postoperative portal-systemic encephalopathy rate is higher in elderly patients [47], and this allows Warren's operation to be proposed even at a relatively advanced age, since it involves numerically reduced encephalopathic complications.

Recognition of general contra-indications for a major operation is, however, more important than the age factor. Patients who are candidates for Warren's operation, as for any other major operation, must be carefully studied from the cardiocirculatory, respiratory, and renal standpoints. In this connection the prognostic and therapeutic usefulness of the systemic haemodynamic staging proposed by SIEGEL [73] (and performed by us in our last 12 patients) in quantifying hyperkinesis should be noted.

Recognition of severe cardiac, respiratory, or renal insufficiency constitutes a contra-indication for the operation, as indeed for any surgery: the patient can be subjected to elective embolization or sclerotization.

Separate reference should, on the other hand, be made to clinical staging of patients, since it allows the hepatic functional reserve and the operating risk to be assessed with good approximation. For prognostic evaluation purposes, Child's classification is the most reliable [12, 32, 76] even if there is discussion as to which individual hepatic function index is of the greatest significance. Like any other shunt operation, Warren's can be performed in stages A and B. In stage C two classes of patients must be distinguished: those belonging to stage C on account of intractable ascites, and those who – albeit with severe impairment of the indices covered by the classification – present with ascites responding positively to medical treatment. In the first group Warren's operation is contra-indicated; in the second group the indication – as for other shunt operations – is uncertain and is based essentially on evaluation of the ratio between the operative risk and expected survival.

Lastly, one special case should be mentioned: the tumoral patient. An untreated current tumor constitutes an absolute contra-indication for the operation, and the same is true for metastasis of an already treated tumor. The operation can, on the other hand, be justified in tumoral patients treated at least

5 years earlier who have no evidence of relapses or metastases, and whose primitive tumor theoretically allows a good percentage of cure.


## Previous Haemorrhage

Certainty of the varicose origin of the haemorrhage is important if the portal hypertension surgery has to retain a prophylactic significance in relation to haemorrhagic *relapses* and not a prophylactic significance in relation to a *possible* haemorrhage.

The known and high frequency of potential bleeding gastroduodenal peptic pathology in cirrhotic patients [41, 42] poses two kinds of problems.

The first and more complex consists in the patient with portal hypertension and associated gastroduodenal lesions observed endoscopically some days after the haemorrhagic episode. Recognition of the previous source of bleeding may be impossible and in any case is always very difficult. It must be remembered that if the source of haemorrhage was an acute gastropathy there may be no endoscopically detectable sign [32] even a short time after the bleeding.

The second kind of problem concerns the patient observed endoscopically during a haemorrhagic episode. Theoretically, the situation is more favourable here, but the possibility exists of mistakenly attributing the real source of bleeding, in a stomach full of blood and coagula, to a gastroduodenal lesion. Hence it is always advisable to repeat the endoscopic examination as soon as the bleeding has stopped.

Absence of absolute certainty as to the source of bleeding poses problems regarding indication for the operation and in respect of treatment.

In this connection we recall the considerations expressed by GALAMBOS [26] on the clinical "dogma" of prophylactic indication: (a) failures of prophylactic operations in patients who had never bled versus conservative therapy have been due to the onset of encephalopathy and hepatic insufficiency; (b) in the trials underlying the "dogma", the prophylactic operations have all been non-selective, and hence theoretically subject to a high encephalopathy rate; (c) utilisation of Warren's operation with prophylactic indication might be conducive to increased long-term survival as compared with conservative treatment, bearing in mind the low encephalopathy rate that this operation involves.

These considerations – when certainty regarding the source of bleeding is not absolute, but when there are nevertheless well-founded clinical reasons for believing that bleeding was due to varices – allow the indication for Warren's operation to be posed with a resonable presumption of not exposing the patient to unnecessary risks.

The coexistence of gastroduodenal peptic ulcer lesions and oesophageal varices that are or have apparently been bleeding imposes the adoption of more complex surgical solutions directed to acting on the peptic lesion as well.

## Anatomical Contra-indications

Anatomical contra-indications to Warren's operation consist in vascular or extravascular conditions that technically prevent performance of the operation. Anatomical contra-indications of vascular type can be divided into those which are detectable pre-operatively and those which are found during operation (the latter will be described in the section on surgical technique).

The former consists in anomalies of formation, patency, diameter, and relations between the splenic vein and the renal vein (Fig. 4). They include conditions – observable angiographically – such as splenic vein thrombosis, splenic vein diameter less than 1 cm, excessive splenic vein shortness, excessive vertical distance between the splenic and left renal veins, and duplication of the left

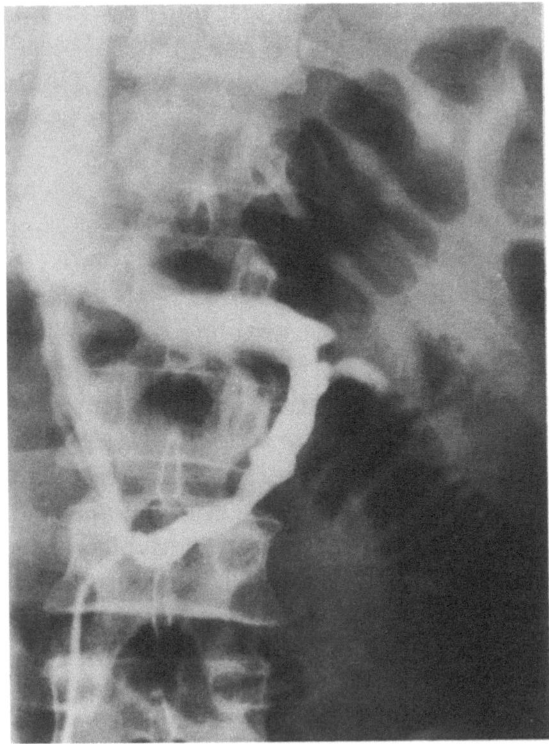

Fig. 4. D. M. (13526/79). Circumaortic renal vein. Catheterization of the retro-aortic branch of the renal vein, with opacification of the whole venous ring

renal vein with long hilus and thin cranial branch [79, 82]. Pre-operative discovery of one of these conditions makes it advisable to adopt alternative surgical solutions.

Anatomical contra-indications of extravascular type consist mainly in conditions that have arisen as a result of previous operations. Warren's operation is not an impossibility in these cases, but surgical access to the splenic and renal veins may be so laborious that it is better to reject the operation from the start.

## Ascites

Pre-operative existence of ascites that is not much reduced or entirely eliminated after adequate medical treatment constitutes a contra-indication for Warren's operation, which, through interruption of the hepatofugal ducts to the varices, involves increased portal pressure only partly offset by loss of the splenic afflux. This pressure increase – although favourable as regards maintenance of hepatic portal perfusion – has an ascitogenic effect [4, 8, 84, 95].

## Hypersplenism

Hypersplenism, defined as a platelet count lower than 100000 and a white cell count of less than 5000, is very frequently associated with portal hypertension, and in its cytolytic and myelo-inhibitory aspects is probably also linked to the stasis that occurs in the splenic pulp. It may therefore be expected that the splenic decompression obtained with Warren's operation, as with other shunts, may have therapeutic effects on the hypersplenism as well [20, 21, 34, 44, 63, 92].

The improvement in the platelet and white blood cell counts after Warren's operation is a fact now fully demonstrated [34] and the presence of hypersplenism does not constitute a contra-indication for the operation, even if there are some opinions to the contrary [67, discussion]. We now exclude from the operation patients who present severe hypersplenism, i. e. with platelet count lower than 30000 and white cell count lower than 2000 (Fig. 5).

## Haemodynamic Contra-indications

The absence or great reduction of hepatic portal perfusion constitutes the only haemodynamic contra-indication for the operation, in the sense that in such

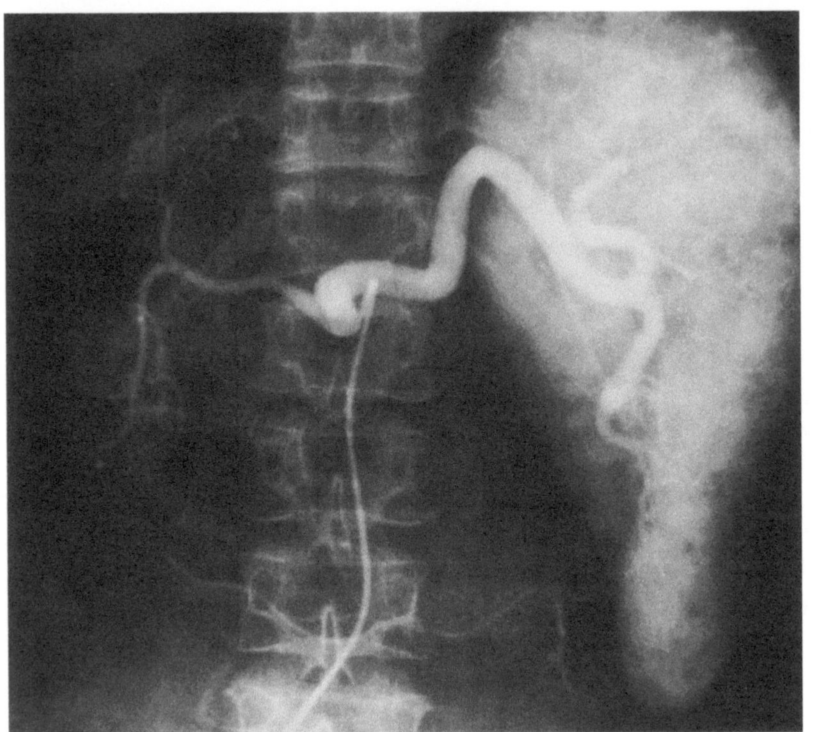

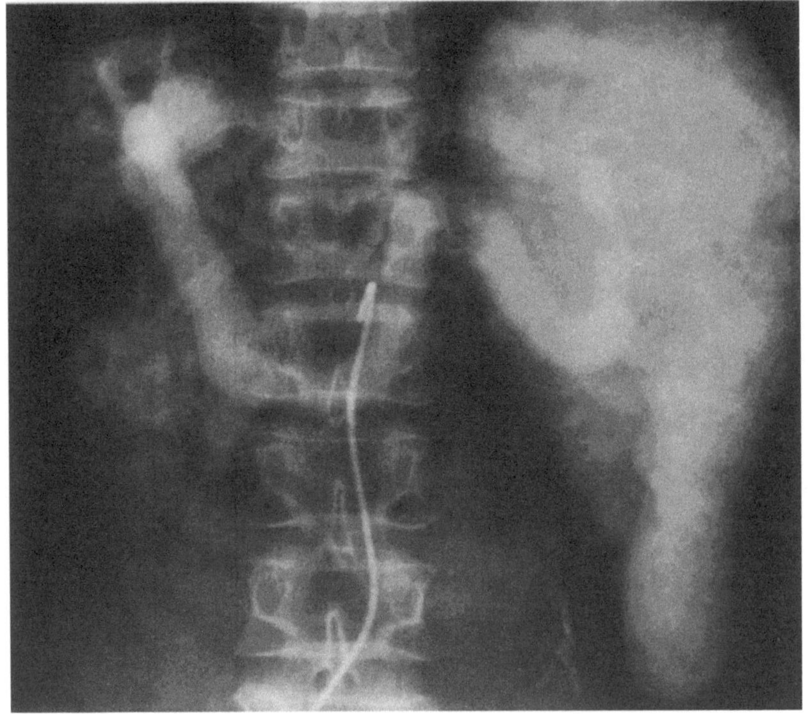

conditions the laborious formation of a distal S-R shunt does not offer advantages as compared with other shunts.

To recapitulate, Warren's operation – as can be seen from all the foregoing considerations – is not automatically applicable to all patients. In fact, among all the candidates for surgical treatment of bleeding oesophageal varices due to portal hypertension, only some can obtain a selective operation. According to ZEPPA [96], only 60% of the candidates can be subjected to Warren's operation; according to our experience, the proportion is around 50%.

**Fig. 5A, B.** Hepatic cirrhosis with considerable splenomegaly. Coeliac arteriogram. **A** Arterial phase. Splenic artery is markedly dilated; hepatic artery and intraparenchymal branches are thin. **B** Venous phase. Considerable increase in volume of spleen. Dilatation of splenic and portal veins. The portal vein is verticalized because of the considerable reduction in volume of the liver

# 4. Preparation for the Operation

Preparation of patients selected for Warren's operation does not present any particular aspect. As always, the problem consists in bringing the patient to optimal hepatofunctional compensation conditions (with particular attention to ascites), and the same for cardiocirculatory, renal and other conditions.

The intensity and length of such care depend on many factors, among which the most important ones are, in our opinion, the date of the last haemorrhage and – in the case of alcoholic cirrhosis – the persistence or cessation of the alcoholic habit. In any case lengthy hospitalization is the best means of adequate preparation for the operation, since the patient can thus be kept at rest and on a strictly controlled diet, with complete abstinence from alcohol [91].

A particular problem consists in the existence of gastroduodenal peptic lesions that have been recognised as not responsible for the bleeding. Their treatment and healing are of great importance in view of the considerable postoperative gastroduodenal haemorrhage rate.

Lastly, preparation for the operation involves careful colon toilet before the operation, as well as protracted pre-operative administration of lactulose, in the endeavour to modify the intestinal bacterial flora and minimise the postoperative encephalopathy risk.

# 5. Technique

The patient is in a supine position, with the left side supported on a cushion. The incision is left subcostal, widened to the whole right rectus muscle. When the peritoneal cavity is opened, attention must be paid to identification and ligation of the umbilical vein, which is often permeable; the ligation is necessary as the umbilical vein can be a means of hepatofugal circulation. After the peritoneum is opened, the abdominal cavity is explored: any adherences hindering access must be carefully ligated, since they are possible sites of postoperative haemorrhage.

The hepatic biopsy, if scheduled, will be performed at this stage of the operation: there will thus be the opportunity to verify haemostasis.

The right gastric vein is ligated and cut; this is followed by skeletonization of the gastric greater curvature, with a section of the gastrocolic ligament as from the pylorus. At this level the right gastro-epiploic vein and any other venous confluents are ligated; this is done in order to disconnect the gastro-epiploic system from the portal axis (Fig. 6). Gastric skeletonization is taken as

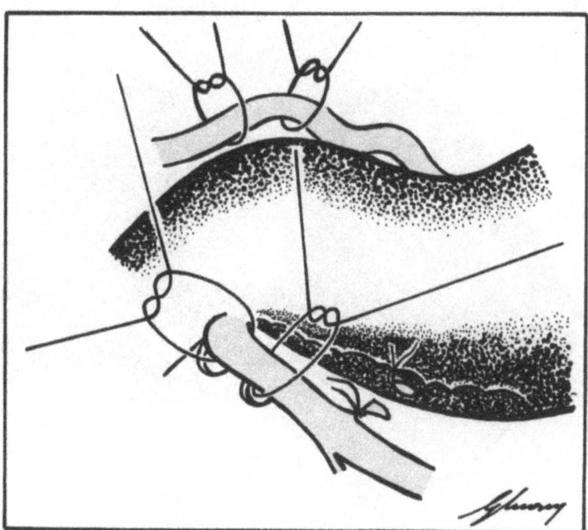

**Fig. 6.** Ligation and section of the right gastric vessels and right gastro-epiploic vessels

far as the level of Mikulicz's point, with respect therefore of the short body-fundus vessels pertaining to the spleen.

Access to the lower margin of the pancreas is thus transgastrocolic (Fig. 7) and not submesocolic as originally indicated [89]. Transgastrocolic access was also suggested by WARREN [91].

We have always preferred transgastrocolic access, made familiar to us by the practice of pancreatic surgery, as it has the following advantages: better access to the retrogastric space; better access to the retropancreatic space; lower risk of colic vascularization damage; exclusion of the duodenojejunal flexure; and better control of haemostasis.

This access may make isolation of the left renal vein more laborious.

After completely freeing the posterior gastric wall from any adhesions, the pancreas inferior margin is isolated, from the mesenteric axis to the tail, and the posterior pancreatic wall is mobilised. At this stage it may be necessary to ligate-cut some small veins running from the peritoneum to the pancreas and/or the inferior mesenteric vein if it has a distal splenic outlet. The pancreas is then surrounded by a tape which, if possible, also includes the splenic artery; in this

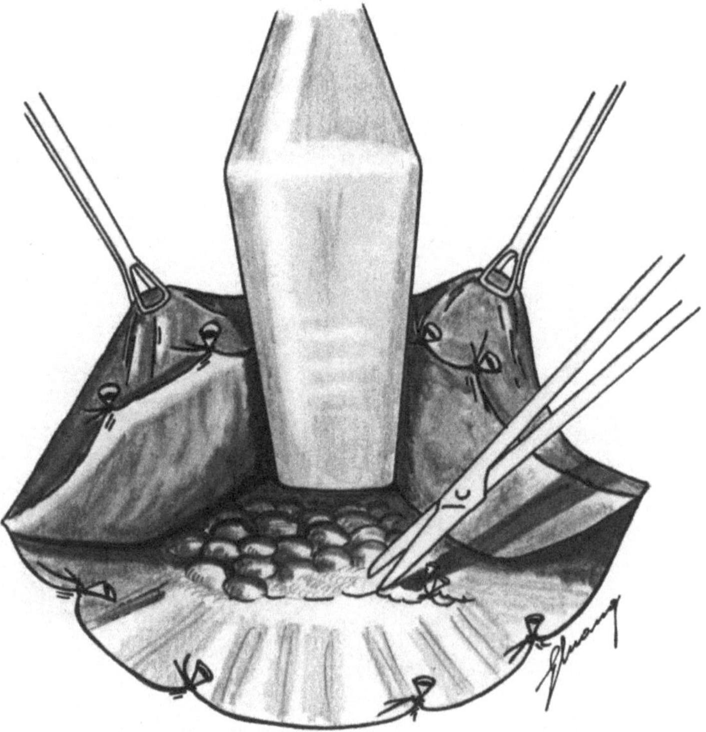

**Fig. 7.** Transgastrocolic access to retrocavity of the epiploons

way, control of any haemorrhage due to tearing of the splenic vein is facilitated. The above handling may be rendered laborious by the presence of chronic pancreatic disease, a not infrequent event in alcoholic cirrhosis of the liver: in our cases there were lesions due to chronic pancreatitis in five cases.

After isolation and raising of the pancreas, the splenic vein is identified first by touch and then by sight; a check is made to ensure that its calibre is as recorded angiographically. Treitz's fascia covering it at the back is incised and cut, and the detachment of the vein from its pancreatic bed is started after ligation and cutting of some hypertrophic lymphatic vessels that sometimes cross the posterior wall of the vein and run on the fascia.

The starting point for detachment is normally the portal confluence, which allows preparation of a venous tract of sufficient length, especially as outlets of small pancreatic veins are rare in this site.

The presence of an inferior mesenteric vein confluent in the splenic vein, which is not very rare (seven cases among our operative subjects), may necessitate ligation of the said vein or starting detachment of the splenic vein as from the inferior mesenteric vein. It should be remembered that Henle's gastrocolic tract and the middle colic vein may also join the splenic vein and that these vessels must likewise be cut in such a case before proceeding to the mobilization of the splenic vein.

The operation may be rendered impossible by the totally intrapancreatic course of the splenic vein (in rare cases). This event – which cannot be foreseen on the basis of the angiographic picture – was found in two of our cases and prevented completion of the operation.

Isolation of the thin-walled [36] splenic vein from the pancreatic bed constitutes the most laborious and stressful part of the operation. The difficulty consists in identifying the pancreatic vessels and ligating them close to the splenic vein (Fig. 8). Normally absent on the antero-inferior margin of the splenic vein, they are concentrated on the supero-anterior wall; their average number is seven. They are short, thin vessels offering low tensile strength and they can easily be torn, especially at the level of their insertion into the splenic vein. Any bleeding therefrom is copious owing to the current portal hypertension and may be difficult to control owing to their position. Their laceration must be corrected solely by suture-ligature of the pancreatic stump and by suture of the splenic breach. The latter operation requires particular attention to avoid stenosis of the splenic vein lumen. Haemostatic attempts by compression or tamponing are always uncertain and ineffective. In this type of haemorrhage NORDLINGER [58] ligates the splenic artery.

The said perforating vessels must be sought and isolated by blunt dissection. A suture-ligature of the splenic end and a ligature of the pancreatic end

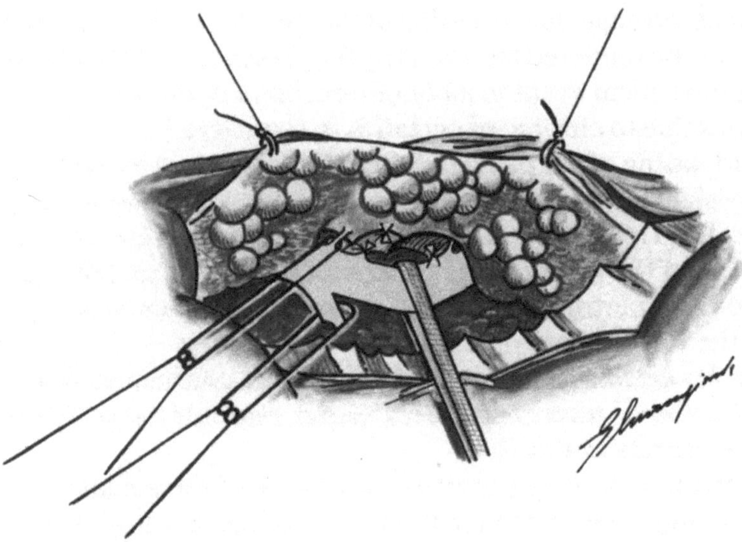

**Fig. 8.** The pancreas has been mobilized. The splenic vein has been isolated from its pancreatic bed. The pancreatic veins and possibly the inferior mesenteric vein are ligated and cut

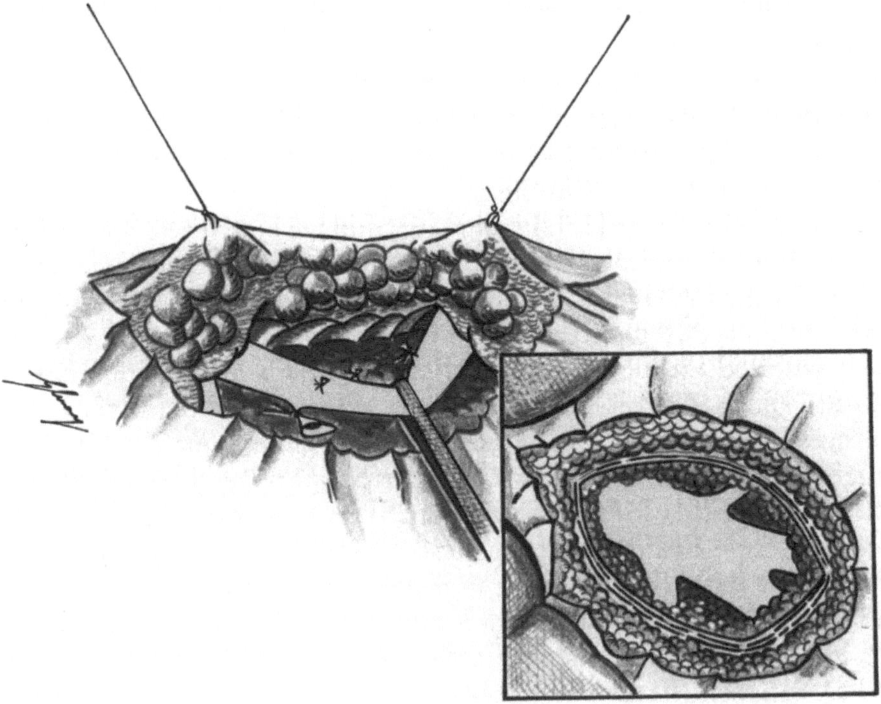

**Fig. 9.** The splenic vein has been mobilized for a sufficient length, starting from its portal outlet. *Inset:* the left renal vein has been prepared from its retroperitoneal bed

will then be carried out; the pancreatic end may also be secured by a metal clip. During location of the pancreatic veins it is advisable to avoid traction of the splenic vein with tweezers; it is safer to surround the vein with a tape and exert delicate traction on the latter.

It is also possible to proceed directly to the distal section of the splenic vein and then to locate the perforating vessels by divaricating the proximal stump; in such cases, however, the left renal vein must be isolated first.

After isolation of the splenic vein for a tract considered sufficient – 5–7 cm – the left renal vein must be identified and prepared (Figs. 9–11).

At this point the importance of pre-operative left renal phlebography must be reiterated, as it will demonstrate both the height of the renal vein in relation to the splenic vein [59] and the existence of any anatomical anomalies (duplication with thin cranial branch, long hilum, retro-aortic course) such as to hinder or prevent performance of the shunt. It must be recalled, in this connection, that interruption of the left renal vein distally to the outlet of the gonadic vein is considered to be devoid of any consequences.

Access to the left renal vein is always hindered by more or less abundant and fibro-oedematous retroperitoneal tissue. The tissue must be sectioned between ligatures in order to avoid troublesome intra- and postoperative lymphorrheas. After identification of the renal vein, it must be isolated and mobilized: mobilization must be ample and such as to allow construction of an anastomosis, not subject to traction, also from the renal sector. Gonadic, adrenalic and plexolumbar vessels converge into the renal vein. They can be cut in order to obtain adequate mobilization of the renal vein; if possible, however, their conservation ensures a further outflow route, particularly when renal pressure is high. Mobilization of the left renal vein may require cutting of Treitz's ligament.

Mobilization of the left renal vein may, especially in obese patients, be very laborious, and may need to be particularly amplified owing to the thickness of the retroperitoneal tissue covering it; the depth of the left renal vein on the frontal planes cannot be seen with phlebography. In some cases the renal vein is so deep that correct anastomosis is possible only through distal section and the construction of a terminoterminal anastomosis or utilization of a vascular graft to extend the splenic vein.

After isolation of the veins, and after compatibility of the relations between the two vessels has been verified, the splenic vein is ligated as close as possible to the portal confluent in order to avoid creation of a cul-de-sac that could become the starting point of a portal thrombosis; for the same reason the portal vein should not be clamped [59]. The splenic vein is then clamped and cut near the ligature, which is secured by a transfixion stitch.

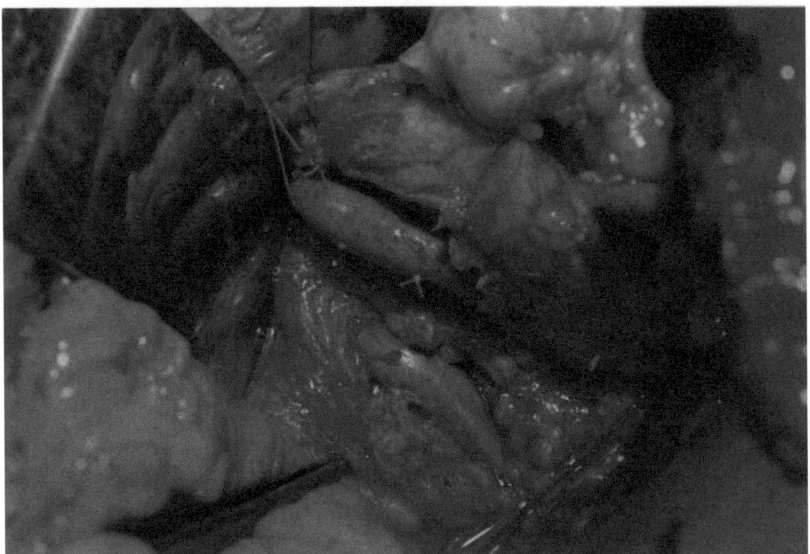

**Fig. 10**

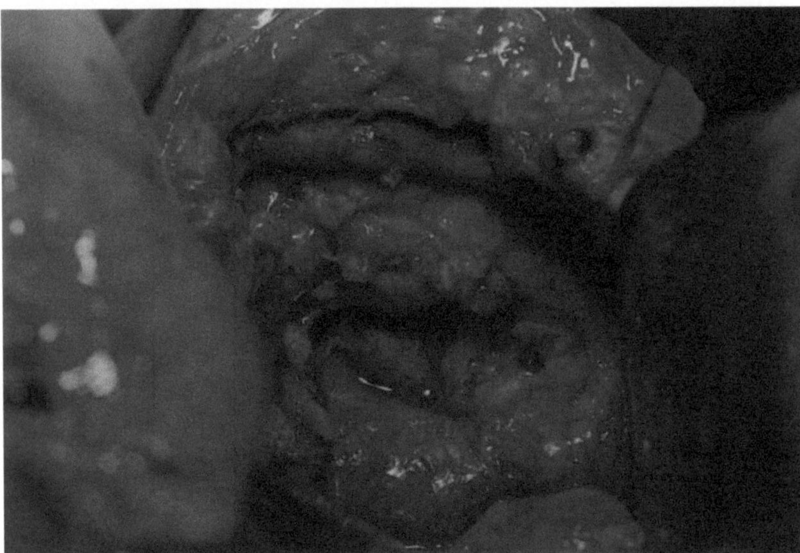

**Fig. 11**

**Figs. 10, 11.** The splenic vein and renal vein have been prepared for anastomosis. It is rare that the relations between the two vessels are as favourable as in **Fig. 10**; generally the left renal vein is covered by a thick wad of fibrous retroperitoneal tissue rich in venous collaterals and lymphatic vessels, as in **Fig. 11**

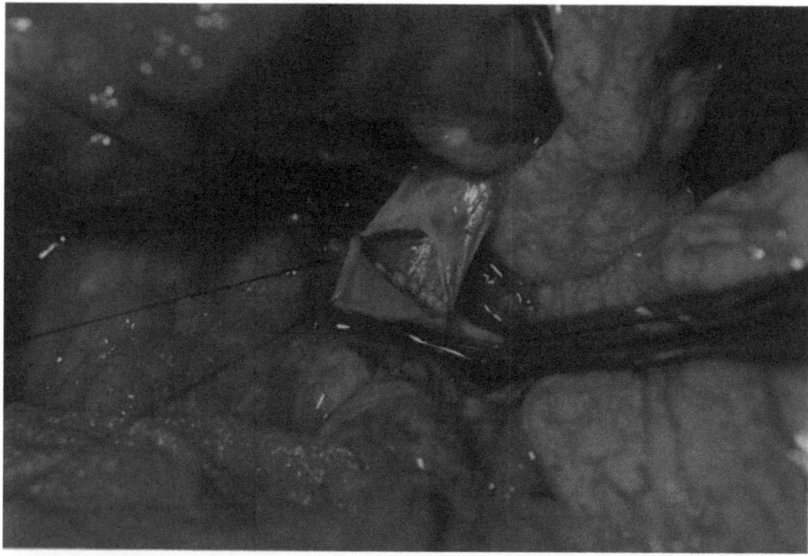

**Fig. 12.** Example of performance of distal splenorenal anastomosis according to Gutgemann's technique

The splenic vein is cut obliquely in order to favour correct angulation of the anastomosis.

The proximal stump of the splenic vein, secured by a bulldog or a vascular clamp, is then brought up to the renal vein. Selection of the point in the vein at which to make the anastomosis is of great importance; positions leading to shunt kinking or twisting must be avoided. With the renal vein clipped tangentially at the selected point, a lengthwise incision is made. In our cases we make a semi-oval incision with dorsal convexity, so as to create an anterior "hatch" [31] (Figs. 12, 13); an elliptical excision of the vein wall can also be made. After fastening the lateral margins of the anastomosis and inserting two traction stitches on the anterior walls of the splenic and renal flaps (which gives better sight of the posterior edges), we suture the posterior wall with a continuous suture of atraumatic thread 5/0[1], starting from the lateral fastening point. The anterior wall is also stitched with a continuous suture, using the thread of the medial fastening point (Fig. 14). Although the suture method originally proposed envisages that the anterior wall is sutured at detached points [91], the method described – due to the hatch incision on the renal vein, which guarantees that the posterior suture is located on a plane lower than the anterior one – has en-

---

1 Angiofil: polyamide monofilament (Lab. Bruneau).

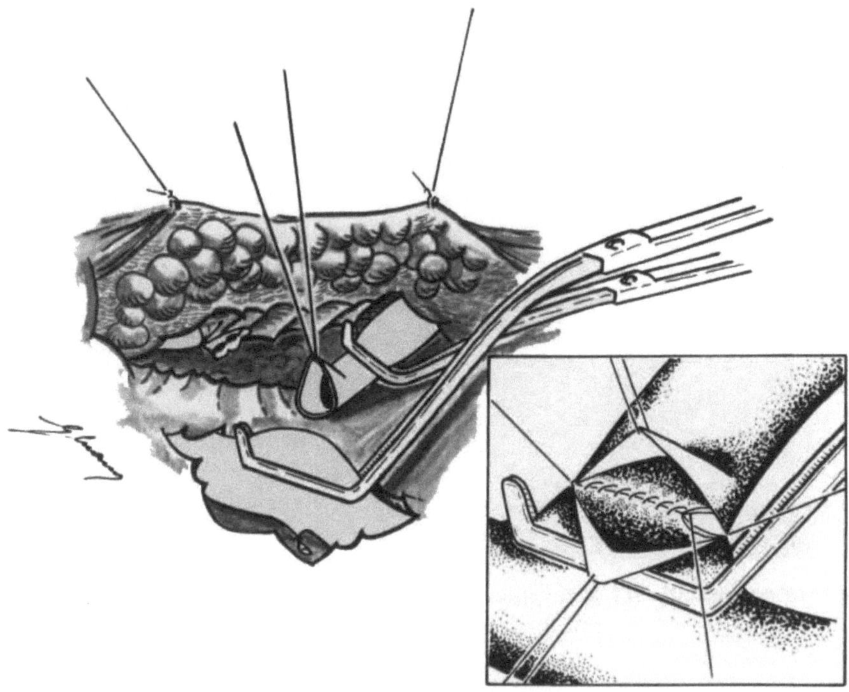

**Fig. 13.** Formation of the distal terminolateral splenorenal anastomosis. The splenic vein has been ligated and cut in the immediate vicinity of its portal outlet. *Inset:* detail of the suture technique, with Gutgemann's hatch

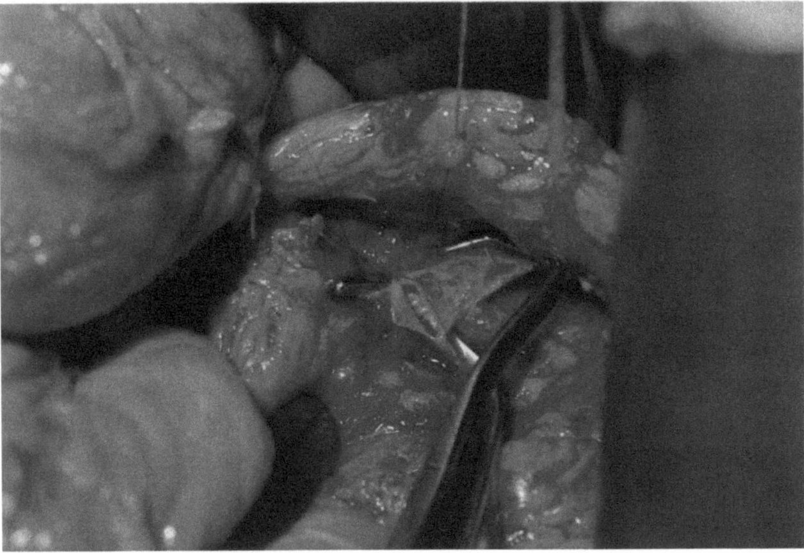

**Fig. 14.** A further example (cf. **Fig. 12**) of performance of distal splenorenal anastomosis according to Gutgemann's technique

sured us a high percentage of anastomotic permeability. The vascular clamps – first the renal and then the splenic clamp – are now slowly released, and the seal of the anastomosis is verified.

The operation is completed by azygos-portal disconnection at the level of the lesser gastric curvature. This is an essential stage for correct performance of Warren's operation, which would otherwise lose its postulated selectivity characteristics (Fig. 15). The gastric devascularization, involving interruption of hepatofugal ducts which may be considerable, is potentially ascitogenic; some surgeons therefore deliberately omit it [4, 8, 56, 85]. In this way, however, Warren's operation is distorted where its selectivity postulate is concerned: the pressure drop induced by the anastomosis cannot fail to favour the establishment of an early hepatofugal circulation. The operation thus altered corresponds haemodynamically to a P-C L-L.

The technical procedures for performance of the disconnection vary in relation to the recognisability of the various anatomotic structures. In other words, only in thin patients will it be possible to recognise and ligate the left gastric vein and any other important venous affluence to the varices under visu-

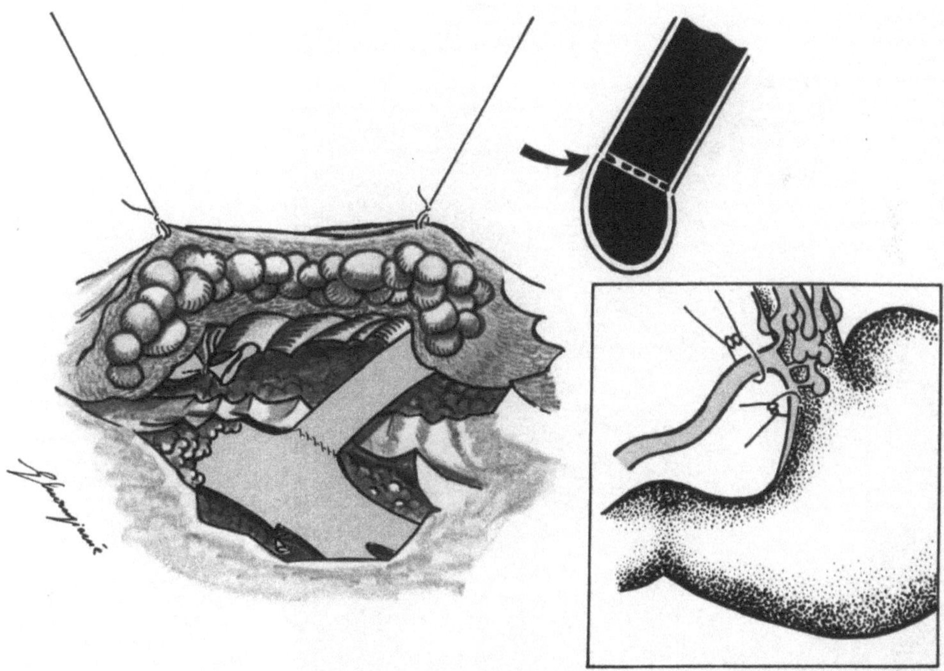

**Fig. 15.** Warren's anastomosis is terminated. The top part diagrammatically illustrates how, with Gutgemann's technique, the suture lines are located on two different planes. *Inset:* ligation of the LGV, an essential stage in Warren's operation

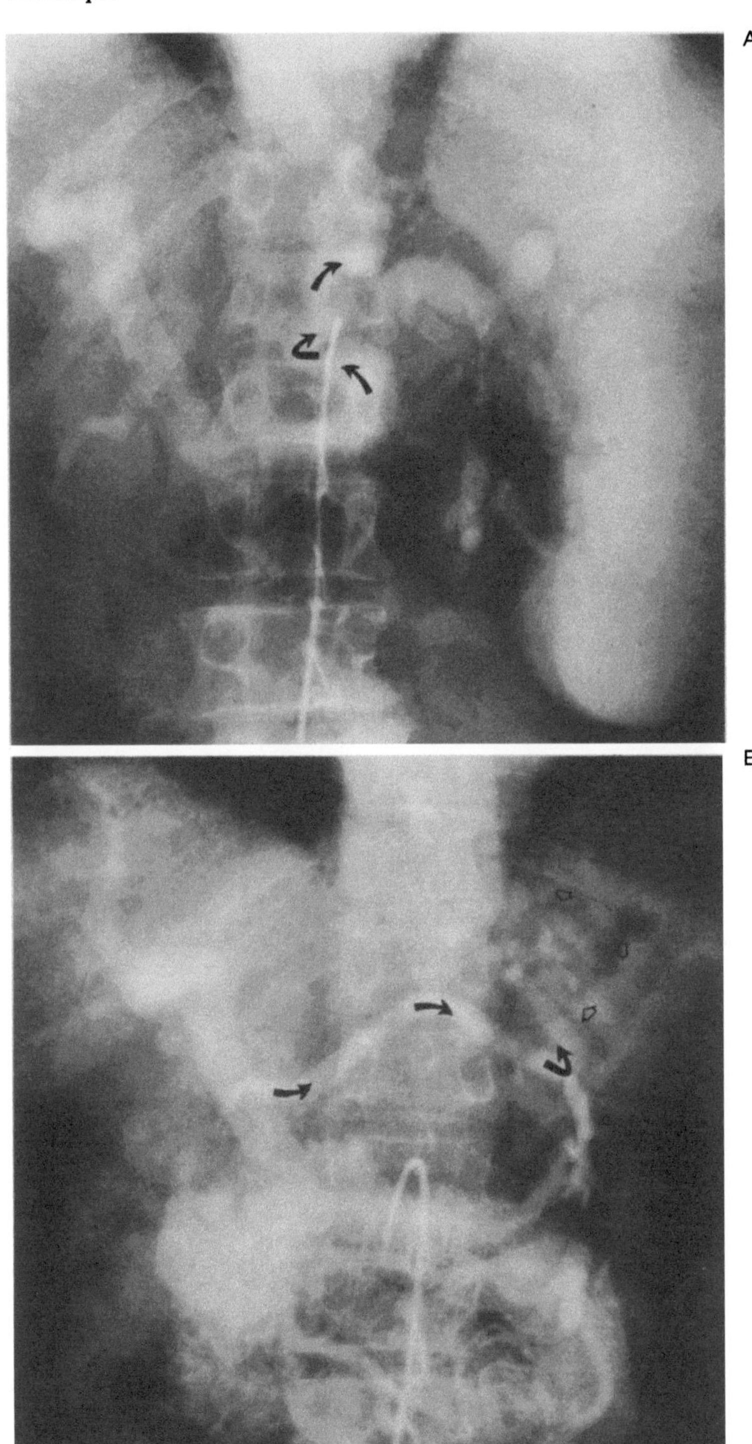

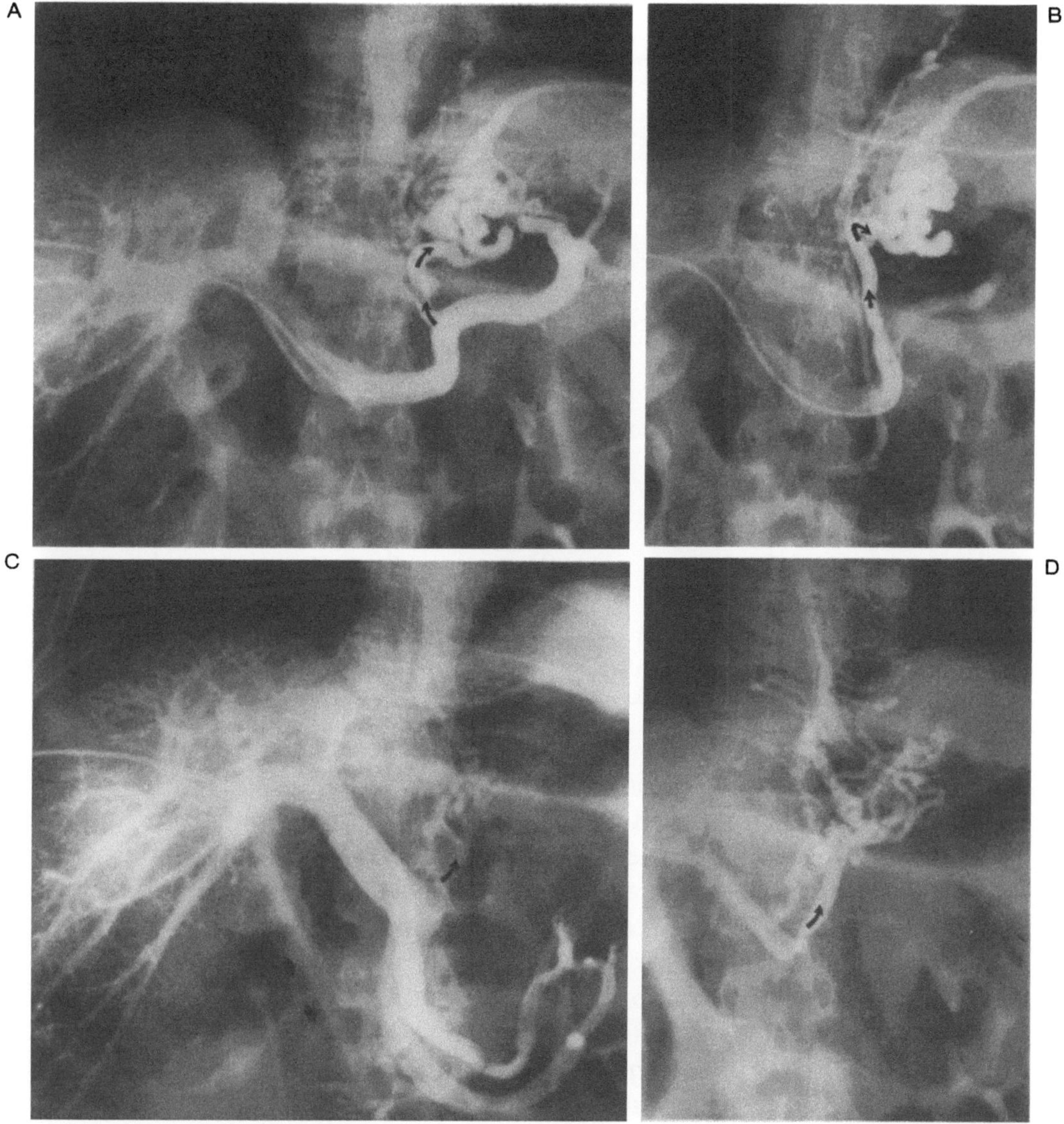

Fig. 17 A–D. Multiple hepatofugal pathways to oesophago-gastric varices. Percutaneous transhepatic portal venography. **A** With injection of contrast medium in splenic vein, visualization of short gastric vein with hepatofugal flow direction *(arrows);* **B** this finding is confirmed by selective catheterization of the gastric branch. **C** With injection of contrast medium in superior mesenteric vein, feeble opacification of left gastric vein, with hepatofugal flow direction *(arrow);* good opacification of umbilical vein *(arrows).* **D** The left gastric vein is much better visualized with selective catheterization

Fig. 16 A, B. B. A. (10431/76). Multiple hepatofugal pathways to oesophago-gastric varices. **A** Splenic angiography. Visualization of left gastric vein, which is noticeably ectasic *(arrows)* and tortuous, originating from the splenic vein. **B** Superior mesenteric angiography. Visualization of dilated right gastric vein *(arrows),* directed to ectasic vein in the gastric fundus *(hollow arrows)*

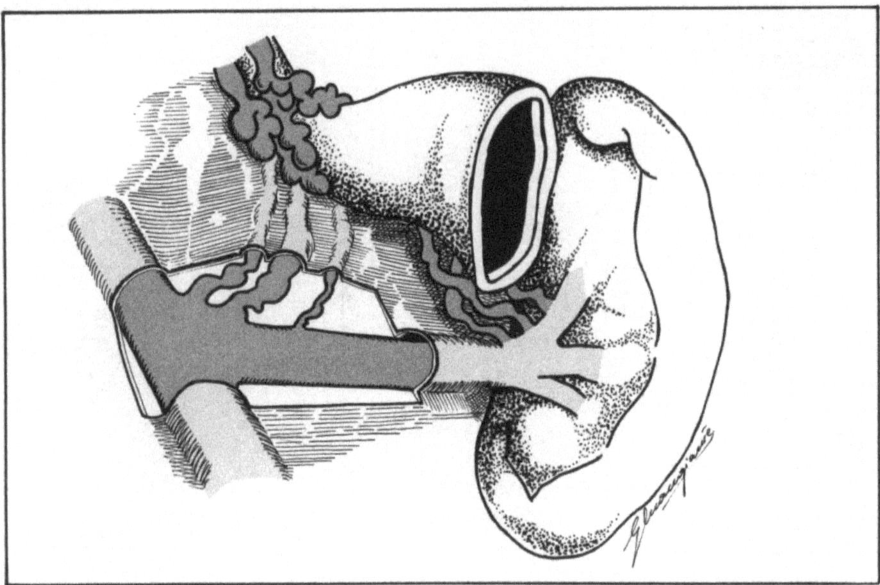

**Fig. 18.** Diagram illustrating the multiple retroperitoneal pathways from splenic and portal trunk to the gastro-oesophageal varices

al control, but this is not the general rule. In the other cases the retroperitoneal thickness does not allow direct visualization of the individual vessels, and it is necessary to proceed first to section of the part of the gastrohepatic ligament and then to carry out devascularization of the fixed part of the lesser curvature as far as the cardias. In these cases it may happen that not only the ascending branch but also the main trunk of the left gastric artery is cut.

The disconnection must be as radical as possible, since the hepatofugal affluences to the varices are often multiple (Figs. 16, 17, 18) as demonstrated angiographically [56, 93]. In this connection it should be recalled that, where there are a number of hepatofugal vessels to the varices, it is not easy to identify the left gastric vein: we term (left gastric vein) LGV the vessel starting from the portal axis, which angiographically appears the most important from the hepatofugal standpoint.

It must also be remembered that it is not infrequent for the LGV to join the splenic vein upstream from the anastomosis. This seems to occur more frequently in portal hypertensive patients, as demonstrated by the recent retrospective research [22] we made on 200 angiographs of portal hypertensive subjects: in 52%, the LGV outlet was in the splenic vein; in 20%, in the porta; and in 28% in the splenoportal junction. Discovery of an LGV – or in any event an important hepatofugal vessel – joining the splenic vein upstream from the anastomosis constitutes, in our opinion, the only contra-indication to ligation of the LGV. Keeping the vessel intact further assists drainage of the varices in the anastomosis. Of course, the remaining vessels must be disconnected [81].

At the end of the operation the anastomosis can be marked with metal clips [14] in order to facilitate radiological identification during postoperative angiography.

We complete the operation by a thin Penrose drainage near to the anastomosis and by layered closing of the abdominal wall.

# 6. Postoperative Treatment

The postoperative treatment does not greatly differ from that commonly used after operations for portal hypertension.

The high capacity of the distal splenorenal shunt makes routine administration of anticoagulants superfluous. In the first 24 h we administer antisludge solutions.

The main problem in postoperative treatment consists in maintenance of a correct hydro-electrolytic balance in the condition of restriction of liquids. The frequent, albeit transient, appearance of ascites in the immediate postoperative period, secondary to interruption of the hepatofugal ducts to the varices, with consequent increase of peripheral portal pressure, means limiting the parenteral water supply to what is strictly necessary.

Prevention and rapid resolution of the ascites are also helped by other measures such as restoration of the oncotically active factors, as well as parenteral administration of anti-aldosteronics and possibly diuretics of furosemide type. Such treatment necessitates electrolytic balance monitoring.

Frequently it is also necessary to administer cardiokinetics with a positive inotropic action, particularly in patients in whom a pre-operative systemic haemodynamic assessment [43, 52, 73] has demonstrated a decompensation or labile compensation condition; it is in this connection that SIEGEL's pre-operative staging reveals all its utility.

Another problem is that posed by the precocious and not infrequent gastroduodenal peptic lesions; whatever their cause, they constitute a concrete danger capable of seriously threatening an otherwise satisfactory postoperative course.

We therefore systematically adopt postoperative cover with $H_2$ blocking agents (Cimetidine), parenterally at first and then orally, maintaining a nasogastric suction tube until completion of canalization.

In all patients we record amylasemia and amylasuria daily, since the appearance of pancreatitic trouble due mainly to the surgical handling of the pancreas is not rare (in fact there is often already an alteration of appearance and consistency of the pancreas during the operation). Discovery of hyperamylasemia and hyperamylasuria requires maintenance of the nasogastric tube for a longer time, as well as aprotinin administration.

On development of the first peristaltic sounds we introduce small enemas with lactulose, which will also be administered orally on completion of canalization.

The Penrose drainage, which acts as sentinel for any bleeding, is removed on the 3rd day.

# 7. Personal Cases

Our cases from 1974 to 1980 cover 42 elective operations. The patients, all with demonstrated previous haemorrhage from oesophageal varices, can be classified as follows: 26 men and 16 women; average age 50 years, with a range from 30 to 67 years. The cases are made up as follows: 26 cases of alcoholic cirrhosis, 9 of posthepatitic cirrhosis, 1 of biliary cirrhosis and 6 of cryptogenetic cirrhosis. All operations were performed in elective conditions after the staging described in the introduction. Nine patients were simultaneously suffering from gastritis, and 11 from duodenitis. In regard to Child's classification, our patients in the immediate pre-operative period belonged to class A (19/42), class B (6/42) and class C (2/42); in 15 of the 42 patients the classification was doubtful. In eight cases the patients had complained of ascites more or less recently; in 11 cases ascites was present at the time of hospitalization, with full regression after pharmacological treatment. There was no severe hypersplenism. The average number of haemorrhages was 70, with an average interval of 24.9 months between the first haemorrhage and the operation. The existence of hepatic portal perfusion was ascertained in all patients; suprahepatic occluding pressures were normal in three patients, while in the other cases it varied between 13 and 37 mmHg, with an average of 25 mmHg. The average pre-operative hospitalization period was 1.8 months. Two operations were performed by venous graft, and three by terminoterminal splenorenal anastomosis [30, 35, 82, 90].

# 8. Results

From the data in the international literature it can be estimated that some hundreds of Warren operations have been performed throughout the world. This is a somewhat tiny fraction of the overall number of shunt operations and could already constitute a difficulty in tracing a profile of the characteristics of the operation. Such characteristics can be analysed from two different standpoints: the first is verification of the theoretical postulates of the operation, and the second consists in the clinical results of the operation.

With regard to the first point, assessment of the validity of the theoretical presuppositions underlying Warren's operation – a validity understood as objective ascertainment of the surgically induced haemodynamic situation – is complex and mainly turns on demonstration of the persistence of hepatic portal perfusion and persistent separation between the mesenterico-portahepatic and oesophagogastrosplenic areas. The problem inherent in this type of evaluation consists in the distinction between effects of the operation and effects of the spontaneous evolution of the cirrhotic liver disease.

As regards assessment of the clinical results according to the usual parameters (mortality, complications, haemorrhagic relapses, encephalopathy), the limited availability in the literature of sets of cases complete from the standpoint of long-term follow-up is a negative aspect. If to this we add the reduced number of randomised trials and the already mentioned difficulty of making a comparison [60] between different sets of cases in which the patients' clinical characteristics and the selection procedures are disparate, it is easy to understand the assertions of those who hold that Warren's operation is not yet fully assessable [48, 77].

## A) Clinical Results

### Operative Mortality

After the already mentioned catastrophic initial operative mortality, the literature reports satisfactory data in this connection, with a maximum rate of 18.5% [38] and with numerous reports of very low operative mortality.

The mean mortality rate can be assessed at around 5%–6% and, if it is borne in mind that this percentage includes emergency operations and operations on unselected patients, it is an acceptable death rate. In particular, WARREN [91] reports a 7% operative mortality; SILVER [74], 5.25%, THOMFORD [83], 0%; NABSETH [56], 11%; ZEPPA [96], 0%; MARTIN [49], 10%; ZEPPA [97], 1.1%; RIKKERS [67], 11.5%; MAILLARD [45], 0%; LANGER [38], 18.5%; BUSUTTIL [11], 11.7%; REICHLE [65], 6% and RESNICK [66], 6%. We had one (2.3%) postoperative death on the 10th day, owing to coma after haemorrhage.

### Postoperative Complications

Non-banal postoperative complications, i. e. those closely linked to the type of operation, consist in ascites, early postoperative haemorrhage and pancreatitis.

The early postoperative appearance of *ascites* is, according to WARREN [87], "the rule". THOMFORD [83] reports 3 cases out of 20; MARTIN [49], 10 out of 50. BUSUTTIL [11] found severe ascites in 41% of his operated patients; NABSETH [56] in 3 of 8; MAILLARD [45] in one patient out of 19 plus one case of chyloperitoneum; and MOSIMANN [53] in 76% of his operated patients. MOSIMANN too reports one case of chyloperitoneum. The appearance of ascites appears to be linked to interruption of the hepatofugal ducts to the varices, with consequent increase in peripheral portal pressure and interruption of the retroperitoneal lymphatics [8]. Ascites tends to spontaneous regression with or without bland pharmacological treatment.

We found postoperative ascites in nine cases, only one of which involved exacting therapeutic problems.

Early postoperative *haemorrhages* are also frequently reported and are, in the great majority of cases, non-varicose in origin and slight [59]; MOSIMANN describes three haemorrhages in 22 operated patients; FUNOVICS [25] reports a 19% rate among his operated subjects.

Haemorrhages of varicose origin do not generally require a further operation and stop spontaneously or with tamponing. The cause of early gastro-duodenal haemorrhages is not known, and moreover it is not easy to make any comparison between their rate after Warren's operation and after other shunt operations.

In our set of cases there were 11 early haemorrhages, of which two were due to gastric ulcer, one to varices, and eight to ulcerative gastritis. Haemorrhage from varices stopped spontaneously.

Postoperative *pancreatitis,* the clinical signs of which were not systematical-ly sought, is typical of Warren's operation owing to the handling that the pancreas undergoes during mobilisation of the splenic vein; however, the episodes are slight and do not reach the clinical picture of necrohaemorrhagic pancreatitis. BUSUTTIL [11] reports postoperative pancreatitis in 20% of cases.

We systematically determined postoperative amylasaemia and amylasuria, finding eight cases of acute pancreatitis.

The rate of early *encephalopathic complications* after Warren's operation finds no significant mention in the literature. In our cases we observed one episode of coma, which was quickly resolved.


## Long-term Mortality

The problem of long-term mortality is perhaps the one that best lends itself to demonstrating the difficulty of making comparisons between the different shunt operations.

Firstly, the randomised sets of cases: RIKKERS [67], after a follow-up of 3–6 years, found 12/23 survivors of Warren's operation as against 17/26 survivors of other, non-selective shunts; LANGER [38] found a long-term death rate of 4/22 after Warren's operation, with a mortality of 9/28 after portacaval shunt – the difference is not statistically significant; GALAMBOS [26] finds that long-term survival after Warren's operation is not statistically significant: there is only a favourable trend versus non-selective shunts.

Isolated reports include the following mortality data: 2 out of 58 (WARREN) [91]; 6.6%, SILVER, (after a follow-up from 4 to 54 months) [74]; 5%, THOMFORD [83]; 12.5%, NABSETH (from 6 to 13 months) [56]; 28%, ZEPPA, (at 5 years, actuarial) [96]; 15.5%, MARTIN [49]; 15.7%, MAILLARD [45]; 13.3%, BUSUTTIL (as against 53.8% for portacaval shunts) [11]; and 25%, REICHLE [65]. SAUBIER [71] has a long-term mortality at 4–42 months of 2 cases out of 23; MOSIMANN [53], 5 out of 19; and RESNICK [66], 4 out of 15 at 1–41 months.

Assessment of long-term mortality cannot fail to take account of the basic cirrhogenic aetiology and the patient's alimentary behaviour. ZEPPA [97], in fact, maintains that after 6 years the mortality in alcoholic patients subjected to distal splenorenal shunt is 89%, whereas in the non-alcoholics it is 39%. ZEPPA also considers that the excellent survival rate in the non-alcoholics demonstrates the functional superiority of Warren's operation over non-selective shunts.

Clearly it is impossible to give any final answer on long-term mortality after Warren's operation for a number of reasons, among which, once again, is the absence of a sufficiently high number of subjects studied for a sufficient length of time, and the difficulty of adapting cirrhotic pathology and its evolution to reliable yardsticks [12, 27, 47, 60, 62].

From the 41 survivors among our cases we are in a position to supply informations on 34, since 7 patients escaped from any form of follow-up. In a period ranging from 6 months to 6 years we observed a long-term death rate of six cases, or 14.6%, broken down as follows: one patient died from hepatic insufficiency due to haemorrhage from gastritis, one from hepatic coma due to haemorrhagic relapse, one from hepatic insufficiency, one from carcinoma of the colon operated 2 years after the Warren operation and two from infarction. We did not find any differences between long-term mortality observed in alcoholic cirrhotics and non-alcoholic cirrhotics (Fig. 19).

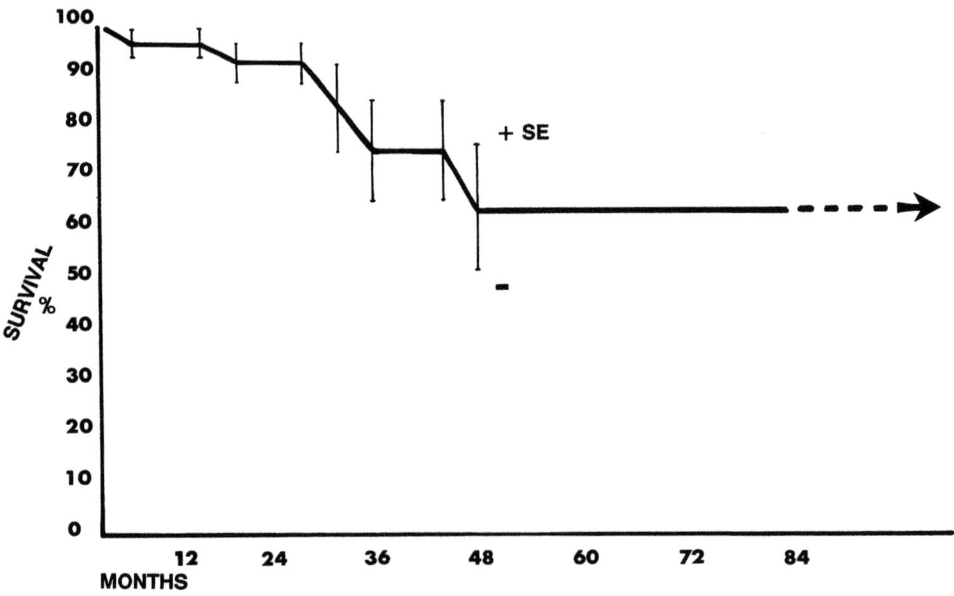


**Fig. 19.** Cumulative survival rate (Berckson-Gage method) of our patients to the beginning of each control interval ± standard error

## Varices – Haemorrhagic Relapses

On the assumption that the aim of shunt operations is not a reduction in the volume of the varices [2], but prevention of haemorrhagic relapses, the reports on the subject appear to demonstrate that after Warren's operation the *persistence of varices* is relatively high. WARREN [91] found persistence of varices in 25%–30% of cases; HUTSON [33] at 1–4 years found the varices to be unchanged in 19% of cases, reduced in 75%, and absent in only 15%; BENACERRAF [3] radiologically found four varices to be unchanged, four to have disappeared, and two to have regressed; SAUBIER [71] endoscopically at 10 days found the varices to be reduced in 17 cases out of 20; MOSIMANN [53] at 15 days found varices to have persisted in 4 out of 17 cases, to have regressed in 7, and to be absent in 6; SILVER [74], without going into details, asserts that long-term radiological controls show that the varices are not consistently reduced.

It must also be recalled that with endoscopic examinations (that we consider 90% precise, while the validity of the barium examination is less) other shunts likewise show a high persistence of varices; DAGRADI [17] asserts that after portacaval shunt it is an exception for the varices to disappear.

*Haemorrhagic relapses* from the rupture of varices seem to have a low incidence after Warren's operation, even though in general the length of the long-term follow-up is less than that for other shunts.

Out of 58 operated cases, WARREN [91] does not report any haemorrhagic relapse due to varices, whereas he reports two relapses not caused by varices. SILVER [74] has one relapse in 16 cases, while THOMFORD [83], with 20 cases, has no haemorrhagic relapses. NABSETH [56], with nine operated patients, reports no relapses from varices, but does report two haemorrhages of non-varicose origin. RIKKERS [67], with 26 operated subjects and with follow-ups from 3 to 6 years, records haemorrhagic relapses in 4% of cases (as against 8% for other types of shunt). LANGER [38] observed two haemorrhages in 27 operated patients at long term, but not of varicose origin; ZEPPA [96], 2 in 66; MARTIN [49], 11 in 42; NORDLINGER [59], 14%, of which one third were due to varices; MAILLARD [45], 0%; SAUBIER [71], 0%; MOSIMANN [53], 2 in 19 and FUNOVICS [25], 5%. HUTSON [33] found haemorrhagic relapses in 2 (3.7%) of 26 patients followed up for 4 years, and BUSUTTIL [11], in 17 operated patients, has no relapses from varices, but one haemorrhage, also not from varices.

Our experience is based on 34 endoscopic follow-ups; we do not take into account the digestive tube radiographs owing to their low significance. In 75% of our cases the varices were much reduced or had disappeared; in 15% they were unchanged, and in 10% they were increased. The average follow-up interval was 19 months, and many patients were examined more than once. The association between thrombosis of the shunt and persistence of varices was not constant [13]; in one case of thrombosis the varices were found to be reduced. There were five *haemorrhagic relapses,* equal to 10.1%, and they occurred at an average interval of 23 months after the operation. We also observed four haemorrhages of non-varicose origin. Our statistics show a significant association between alcoholic aetiology, continuing abuse and haemorrhagic relapse.

## Hepatic Function

The data on the postoperative trend of the hepatic function and the long term ones are not very abundant. However, we can report works by SILVER [74], who assesses the stability of hepatic function indices, and GALAMBOS [26], who finds the MRUS trend significantly in favour of Warren's operation when compared with the mesentericocaval shunt. RIKKERS [67], comparing Warren's operation with other shunts in a randomised trial, found that early controls showed that the MRUS trend and common indices (Child) were more favourable to a statistically significant extent after Warren's operation. RIKKERS also – after a follow-up of 3–6 years – finds that MRUS and Child's indices are still better in the subjects operated on with a distal splenorenal shunt, but no longer to a statistically significant extent, unless for both groups the permeable shunts only are taken into consideration; if this is done the differences are again significantly in favour of the former.

In all 34 of our followed-up patients, the common hepatic function indices (not including MRUS) were frequently determined. The results, still with an average interval of 19 months, can be summarised as follows: one case of thrombocytopenia; four cases of severe impairment of the hepatic function indices; and in the remaining patients, stationary hepatic function indices.

## Encephalopathy

This is the aspect of Warren operation's clinical results that is less open to discussion; in fact its superiority in avoiding long-term encephalopathic complications is almost unanimously recognised. We must, however, mention that in the literature the procedure for diagnosis and quantification of the encephalopathy is often not reported, nor are the details of pre-operative encephalopathy available. It should be recalled that SILVER [74], with a follow-up of

2–28 months, did not find encephalopathy in any of the followed-up patients and observed that ammonemia drops from an average of 95 mg% in the pre-operative period to an average of 77 mg% in the long-term follow-ups. NAB-SETH [56], at 6–13 months, found no case of encephalopathy among his controls, and subsequently [57] found 1 case of encephalopathy among 12 operated patients. GALAMBOS [26] found that the lower encephalopathy rate after Warren's operation as compared with after mesentericocaval shunt is statistically significant. RIKKERS [67], with a follow-up of 3–6 years, found a 12% encephalo pathy rate after Warren's operation, as compared with 52% for other shunt operations; the difference is statistically significant. REICHLE [65], in a controlled prospective study, found that Warren's operation is superior to mesentericocaval shunts as regards the encephalopathy rate to a statistically significant extent. BUSUTTIL [11] found the lower encephalopathy rate after Warren's operation significant in comparison with other, non-selective shunts. LANGER [38] found three cases of slight encephalopathy among 22 patients subjected to Warren's operation versus 14 cases (5 of which were severe) among 28 patients subjected to portacaval shunt; the difference is statistically significant. Other reports are by WARREN [91], with 2 encephalopathies out of 58 cases; THOMFORD [83], with 1 coma out of 28 cases; MARTIN [49], 18%; MAILLARD [45], 2 encephalopathies of slight severity among 19 operated patients; SAUBIER [71] no encephalopathy up to 42 months; NORDLINGER [59], 3.7% encephalopathy against 50% in controls; MOSIMANN [53], 1 out of 19; FUNOVICS [25], 6% of severe encephalopathies and RESNICK [66], with 25% of encephalopathies, half of which were severe.

Our 34 patients were observed by means of EEG, ammonemia determination, neurological assessment and aptitude evaluation in regard to usual working activity. We observed EEG changes only in the patient who had postoperative coma. Ammonemia remained constant with the sole aid of dietary measures – with or without lactulose – in 23 of the 28 long-term survivors. In these 23 patients the neurological conditions and work aptitude can be considered good. In the other five patients (three of whom were alcoholics) medium-severe encephalopathy is present.

## B) Haemodynamic Results

In this section no account will be taken of the results of modified operations, i. e. those distal splenorenal shunts in which the disconnective stage is deliberately omitted on the grounds of wishing to avoid ascitic complications. These are ample sets of cases excellently documented from the pre- and postoperative angiographic standpoint [8, 56, 84, 85, 93, 94].

The summarised results document a high percentage of patency of the anastomosis, and progressive reduction of the portal hepatic perfusion as a result of hepatofugal vessels of increasing size directed to the shunt mainly through the varices. Even if, as we shall see, the haemodynamic results of the modified operations do not greatly differ from those of the selective operations, the a priori rejection of the selectivity criterion automatically excludes them from this discussion.

The main postulated aims of Warren's operation consist in effective prevention of haemorrhagic relapses and an increase in long-term survival with lower encephalopathy, and this is to be obtained through maintenance of portal perfusion and, to a lesser extent, absence of hepatofugal phenomena through surgical separation between the portal-mesenteric area and the oeseophago-gastro-splenic area. Warren's operation is capable of ensuring effective prevention of haemorrhagic relapses due to oesophageal varices, with a significantly lower encephalopathy rate as compared with "total" shunts.

Are these better results justified, in line with the starting hypothesis, by the postulated haemodynamic characteristics?

Haemodynamic assessment appears essential in an operation conceived according to haemodynamic criteria, but the literature has little to say in this respect [77]. The asserted roughly 90% maintenance of portal hepatic perfusion [91] reported by WARREN has not proved to be so frequent. The *intra-operative observations* have already demonstrated that the shunt in itself immediately induces a drop in portal pressure [45]. According to MAILLARD, who used manometric and flow-metric procedures, while no significant variation in the shunt flow is recorded after disconnection, there is a $56 \pm 18\%$ mean drop after splenic artery clamping, reflecting the potential of shunt hepatofugal flow [18, 28]. MAILLARD likewise recorded a reduction in total hepatic blood flow (THBF) from $1250 \pm 475$ ml/min to $790 \pm 40$ ml/min, comparable to what is recorded after terminolateral portacaval shunt; the mean shunt flow after Warren's shunt is equal to that of non-selective operations.

MATHJÊ [52], on the other hand, who intra-operatively adopts Krypton 85 extraction, did not find portal hepatic perfusion variations after shunt.

It must, however, be recalled that the validity of intra-operative recordings is limited by narcosis and by the opening of the abdominal wall [72].

On the other hand, in regard to more reliable *haemodynamic assessments,* obtained in conscious patients by transhepatic catheterization of the portal vein, WIDRICH's work [94] is to be quoted. However, WIDRICH based his findings on only three cases at a little more than 2 years after the operation and reported a considerable portal perfusion drop, with flow inversion in one case. In one case the same author records a nearly fourfold increase of splenic vein flow. REICHLE [64], in a case observed 7 days after the operation by means of omphaloportal manometry, observed a portal pressure drop from 39–41 to 22–25 cm $H_2O$.

Using extractive methods BENACERRAF [3], 15 days after the operation, observed a significant reduction in THBF in 11 cases (from 1.19 litres/min to 0.84 litres/min on average).

With *suprahepatic manometry* BENACERRAF found no significant variations of the pre- and postoperative pressure gradient in 13 patients. With hepatic manometry NORDLINGER [59] found signs of flow inversion in 40% of cases.

With regard to *angiographic tests,* which are relatively more fully reported in the literature, the main information concerns portal perfusion, hepatofugal circulation, shunt thrombosis, portal thrombosis, and variations in the size of the splenic artery, hepatic artery, splenic vein, and spleen. It should be remembered that angiography is, however, capable of supplying only a rough quantitative estimate [67].

Our cases consist of 27 patients observed angiographically; 13 were tested only once; 13, twice; and 1, three times, making a total of 42 angiographic readings.

The observations were made from 1 to 63 months after the operation, with an average of 14 months. This mean value becomes 21 months if only the maximum interval between operation and last angiographic test is considered. Taking only the 14 patients with more than one angiographic reading, it can be observed that the first reading was made after 6.5 months on average, the second after 31 months, and the third after 44 months.

The angiographic study always consisted in selective arteriography of the coeliac trunk and the superior mesenteric artery; superselective catheterization of the splenic artery and hepatic artery was also frequently used. In 16 patients selective catheterization of the shunt was likewise attempted, with success in 12 cases.

The WHVP was determined only occasionally.

The following parameters were evaluated: (a) patency of the anastomosis; (b) spleen volume; (c) splenic artery and vein diameters; (d) portal vein diameter, portal flow direction, and characteristics of any hepatofugal circulations and (e) liver dimensions and arterial vascularization. The results of the angiographic test or tests were compared with the pre-operative angiographic picture.

## Portal Perfusion

Maintenance of hepatic portal perfusion is the prime aim of Warren's operation. It is therefore logical that particular interest should be directed to observation and evaluation of this fundamental factor (Fig. 20).

Only 15 days after the operation BENACERRAF [3] demonstrated a constant portal flow reduction in 19 patients with portal perfusion absent or low in 3 out of 14 patients who had a medium or considerable perfusion prior to the operation. In three observations made at 6–12 months he noted a further reduction in portal diameter.

NORDLINGER [59], on the other hand, followed up 89 patients who had undergone Warren's operation (66 within 6 months, and 23 up to more than 5 years) and 49 non-selective shunts. In the tests made within 6 months he found portal perfusion to be present in 88% of the selective shunts (as against 0% of the non-selective shunts, with a statistically significant difference). The extent of the flow remained unchanged in 81% of cases. In the late tests the hepatoportal flow was present in 70% of cases (and the difference versus the controls is still statistically significant). NORDLINGER does not, however, give figures on portal diameter reduction.

BUSUTTIL [11], who followed up 30% of 17 operative patients for up to 20 months, found, on the other hand, that the hepatopetal portal flow is constantly maintained.

RIKKERS [67], in a randomised study covering 26 Warren operations versus 29 non-selective operations, found in the early tests that the more frequent presence of portal hepatic perfusion after Warren's operation (14 out of 16 vs 2 out of 20) is statistically significant, whereas after 3–6 years, although the difference persists, it is no longer statistically significant (in 58% of cases no portal hepatic perfusion is evidenced).

SAUBIER [71], observing 20 patients at 10 days and again at 2 months after the operation, found portal perfusion to be present in 18 out of 19 patients. FUNOVICS [24] finds portal circulation to be present only hepatopetal in 33% of cases, with total flow inversion in 8.3% of cases.

In our tests the portal vein flow retained its *hepatopetal direction* in 22 out of 23 patients with patent shunt (95.6% of the patent shunts), with a *reduction in portal vein diameter* in 20 out of 23 patients (86.9% of patent shunts), with a decrease from a mean diameter of 1.73 cm (minimum 1.2, maximum 2.2) to a mean diameter of 1.16 cm (minimum 0.4, maximum 1.9)[2]. The portal diameter reduction was observed both at the early and late tests (Figs. 20, 21, 22). In one

---

2 $t = 4.905$, $P < 0.001$, highly significant

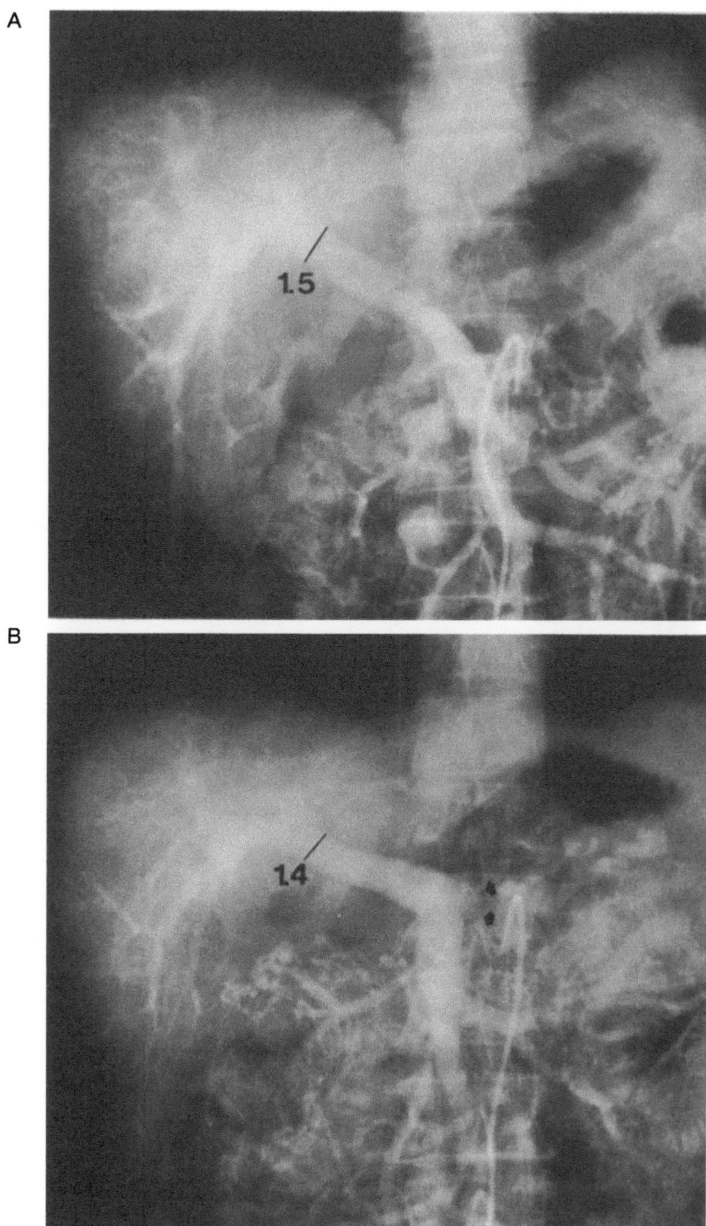

**Fig. 20 A, B.** P. C. (6754/78). Changes in portal circulation.
**A** Pre-operative angiography. Portal vein with diameter of 1.5 cm. No hepatofugal circulation is evident.
**B** Postoperative angiography (24 months). Slight reduction in diameter of portal vein (1.4 cm), without evidence of hepatofugal circulations. Visualization of short stump of splenic vein, ligated close to the splenomesenteric confluence *(arrows)*

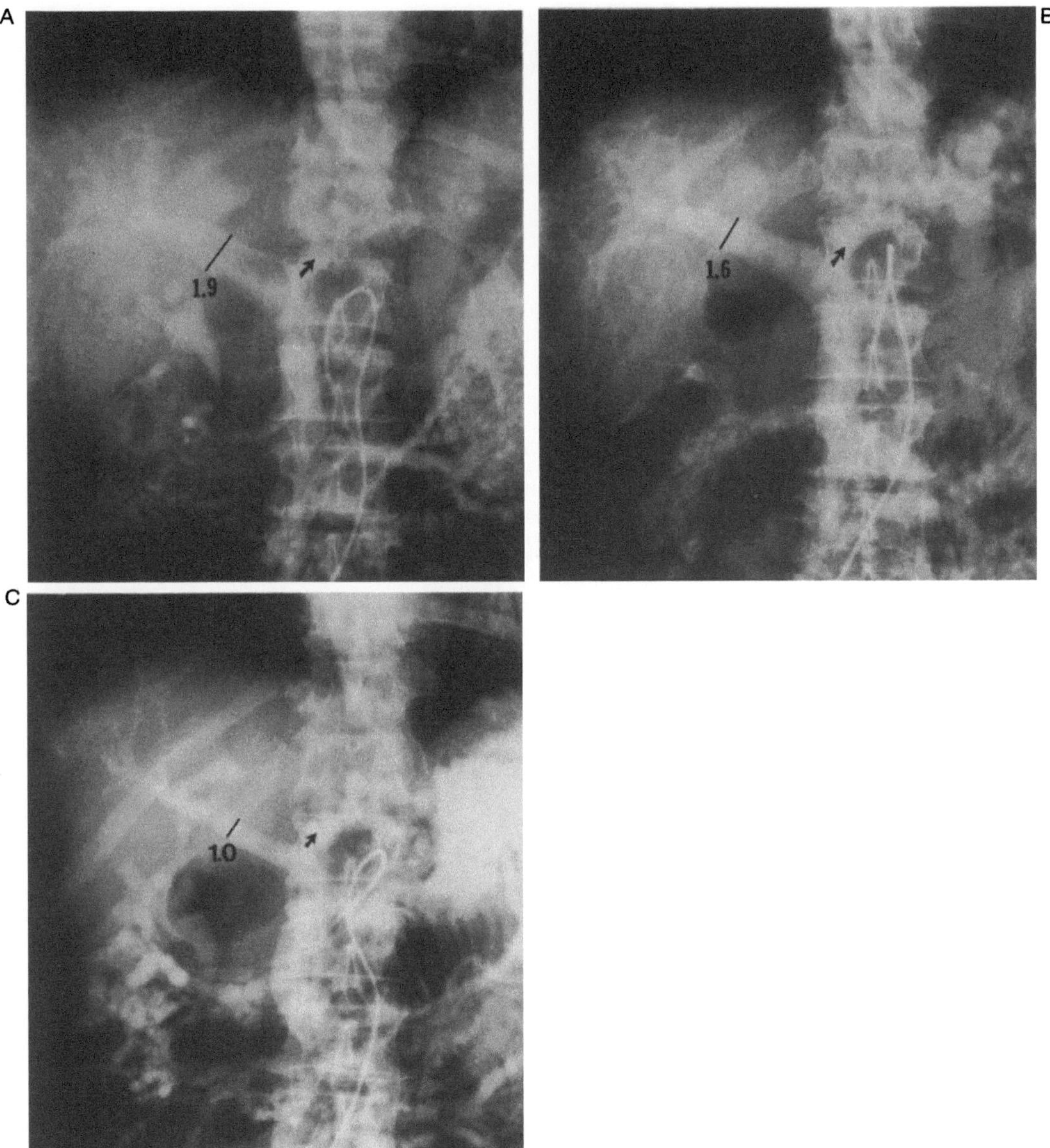

**Fig. 21 A–C.** P. F. (14556/77). Changes in portal circulation.
**A** Pre-operative angiography. Portal vein with diameter of 1.9 cm. Hepatofugal flow through large left gastric vein *(arrow)*. **B** Postoperative angiography: first follow-up (1 month). Reduction in diameter of portal vein (1.6 cm). Persistence of hepatofugal flow through left gastric vein *(arrow)*. **C** Postoperative angiography: second follow-up (28 months). Further marked reduction in diameter of portal vein (1 cm). Retrograde filling of left gastric vein is still present *(arrow)*. Dilated veins can be observed in ascending colon site

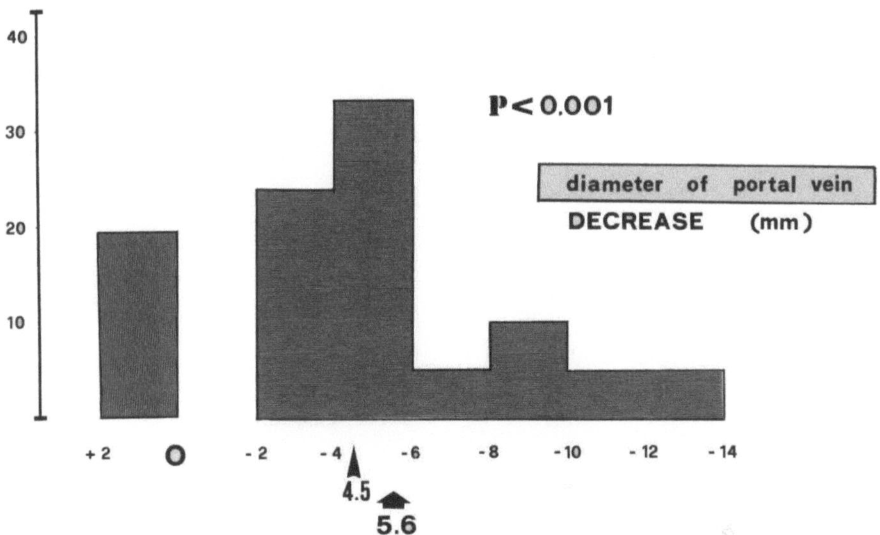


**Fig. 22.** Variations (expressed in millimeters) in the diameter of the portal vein after distal S-R shunt. On the first angiographic control (performed after a mean interval of 6.5 months from the operation) we found a mean decrease of 4.5 mm *(small arrow),* while on repeated controls (performed after a mean interval of 31 months from the operation) we found a mean decrease of 5.6 mm *(large arrow).* The postoperative decrease is statistically significant at the 0.001 P level

of the patients with retained hepatopetal flow a *partial thrombosis of the portal vein* was observed (2 months after the operation) (Fig. 23); in another patient, *complete thrombosis* of the portal vein was observed after 16 months, with development of portal cavernoma with hepatopetal direction of the mesenteric blood flow. In one patient out of 23 (4.3%), *portal flow inversion* was observed 35 months after the operation. The reduction in portal diameter was progressive over time (Fig. 24).

*Portal thrombosis* is observed with considerable frequency and is attributed to intra-operative traumas. It is a complication which, if total, invalidates the aim of maintenance of portal perfusion. Thromboses are reported by NORDLINGER [59], who found complete portal thromboses in 3.5% of cases and partial thromboses in 13.8%. ROTSTEIN [69] found five thromboses in 48 tests, and BUSUTTIL [11], 1 in 17 tests. LANGER [38] found portal thromboses in 11.1% of cases, while SAUBIER [71] found total thromboses in 5% and partial thromboses in 31.5%. RIKKERS [67] found thromboses in 12.5% of cases; NABSETH [56], 1 thrombosis in 12 cases and MAILLARD [45], 1 thrombosis in 12 cases.

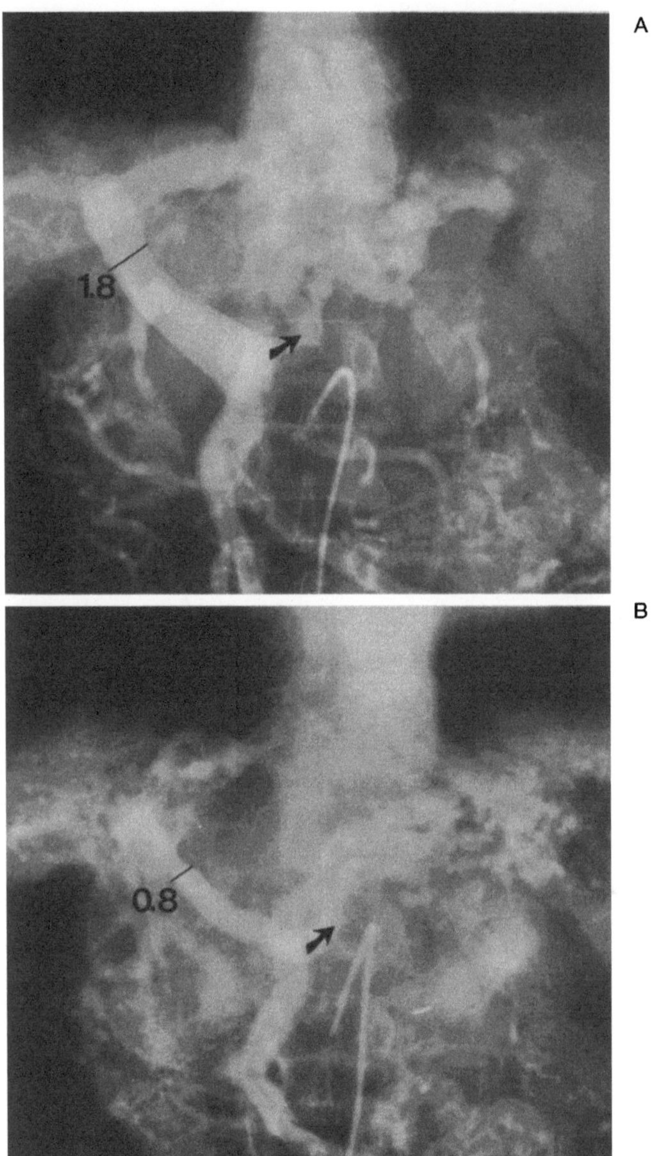

**Fig. 23 A, B.** C. O. (18447/77). Changes in portal circulation. Portal vein thrombosis.
**A** Pre-operative angiography. Portal vein with diameter of 1.8 cm. Hepatofugal flow through dilated left gastric vein *(arrow)*.
**B** Postoperative angiography (2 months). Partial thrombosis of portal vein, which shows reduction in diameter (0.8 cm) and non-homogeneous opacification. Hepatofugal circulation is still evident *(arrow)*

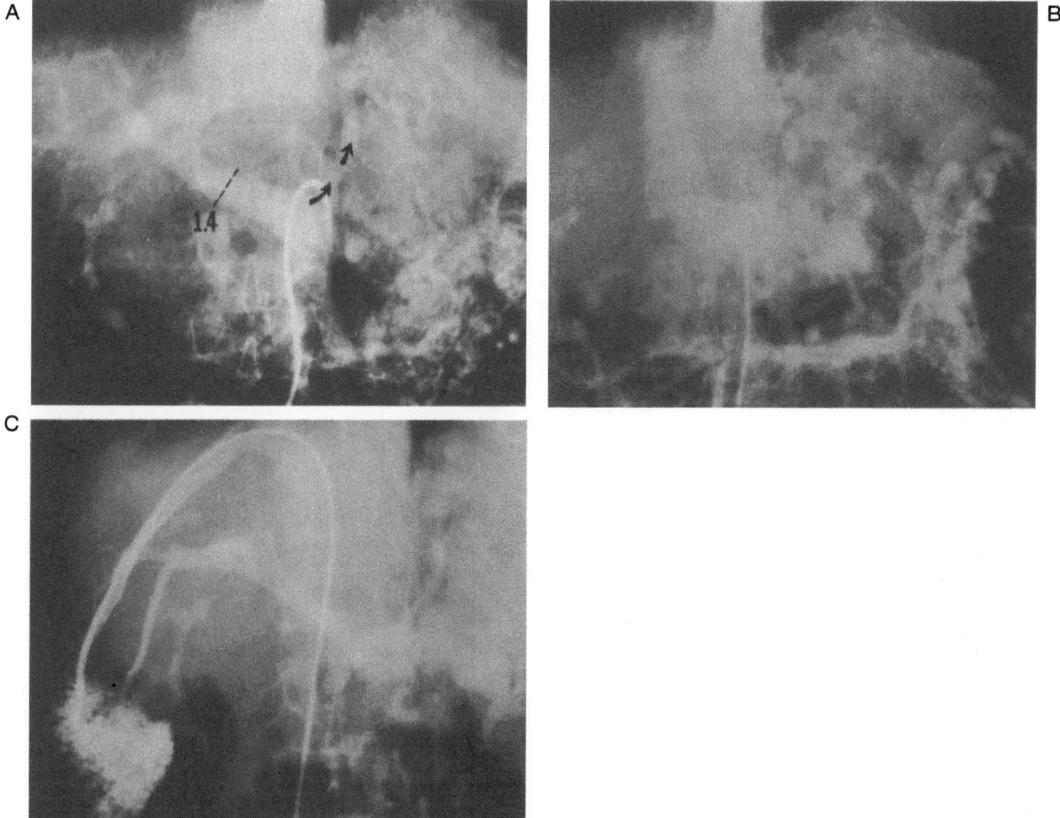

**Fig. 24 A–C.** R. A. (2752/73) Changes in portal circulation.
**A** Pre-operative angiography. Hepatopetal flow in the portal vein with diameter 1.4 cm; hepatofugal circulation through left gastric vein *(arrows)*.
**B, C** Postoperative angiography (34 months). **B** In the venous phase of superior mesenteric angiography the portal vein is not opacified. Blood flow takes place through multiple collaterals, with good opacification of anastomosis and inferior vena cava. (**B**) Wedged hepatic venography demonstrates hepatofugal flow in the portal vein with feeble opacification of the collateral pathways visualised in **B**

## Hepatofugal Pathways

Another very important factor in haemodynamic evaluation is postoperative angiographic demonstration of hepatofugal collateral pathways, the presence of which after Warren's operation is attributed on the one hand to the practical impossibility of completely disconnecting the mesenterico-portal-hepatic circulation from the gastro-oesophago-splenic circulation [45], and on the other to

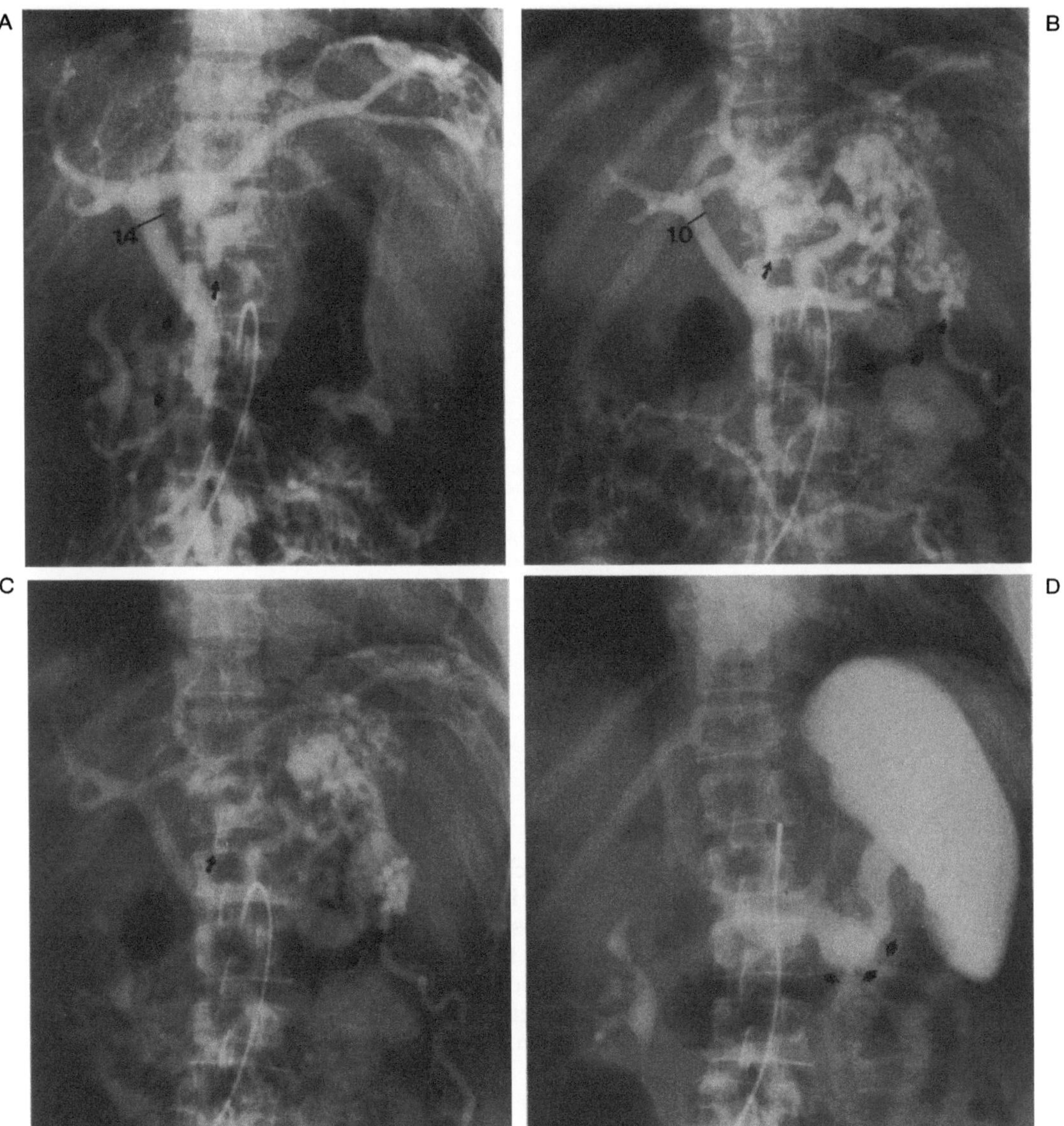

**Fig. 25 A–D.** L. M. (913/80). Changes in portal circulation.
**A** Pre-operative angiography. Portal vein with diameter of 1.4 cm. Hepatofugal flow through umbilical vein *(arrows),* dilated left gastric vein *(arrow),* and pericardiophrenic veins. **B–D** Post-operative angiography (5 months). In the venous phase of the superior mesenteric angiography **(B, C)**, marked reduction in diameter of the portal vein (1 cm). Hepatofugal flow through left gastric vein is still evident *(arrow);* development of hepatofugal circulation through short gastric vein and dilated mesocolic veins, with good opacification of splenic vein and anastomosis *(arrows,* **B, C***).* Confirmation of anastomosis patency in the venous phase of splenic angiography **(D)**

the spontaneous development of intrahepatic resistances, while resistances in the splenic area are diminished (Fig. 25).

BENACERRAF [3] found hepatofugal circulation in 11 out of 19 patients tested within 15 days; in 3 patients at the long-term follow-ups there was an increase in the hepatofugal circulation. According to this author the disconnection is ineffective in the majority of cases at 15 days, and in all at the long-term follow-ups.

SAUBIER [71] finds eight cases of hepatofugal circulation to the varices among his 19 tests.

According to NORDLINGER [59], 25% of patients with residual varices evidenced endoscopically do not show hepatofugal collaterals in the abdominal angiography; he asserts that demonstration of these flows is frequent after distal splenorenal shunt and that their frequency increases as time passes.

Among our cases hepatofugal pathways were recorded in 20 out of 23 patients with a patent shunt (86.9%); the hepatofugal circulations were directed to the gastric fundus (Fig. 26). More rarely, and especially in the late follow-ups, a second hepatofugal route was evidenced through the veins of the greater omentum and the mesocolon, and directly joining the splenorenal shunt (Fig. 27). The increase in hepatofugal pathways was found to be progressive over time. In the three patients (at 5, 9, and 24 months after the operation) in whom no hepatofugal pathways were evidenced, reduction in portal diameter co-existed in two, while in the third the portal diameter was unchanged as compared with before the operation.


## Patency of the Shunt

Demonstration of patency of the shunt is another subject of fundamental importance, especially in view of the clinical consequences that thrombosis may involve; in fact a state of local hypertension is created in this way [39, 70] (Fig. 28).

According to WARREN [91], the demonstration of patency is successful in nearly all cases (55 out of 58); THOMFORD [83], in fact, reports 100% patency in 18 cases, as do BUSUTTIL [11] in 17 tests, BENACERRAF [3] in 20 cases and SAUBIER in 20 cases (with one stenosis of the anastomosis), as well as FUNOVICS [24].

BERCHTOLD, on the other hand [5], found occluded shunts in 50% of cases, and RIKKERS [67], in 10% (versus 18% in the non-selective shunts). NABSETH [56] found two occluded shunts in 12 cases, while NORDLINGER [59] found thromboses of the anastomosis in 9% of cases, versus 26% of thromboses in the non-selective shunts; 6.7% of thromboses are already recorded at the early tests. Ac-

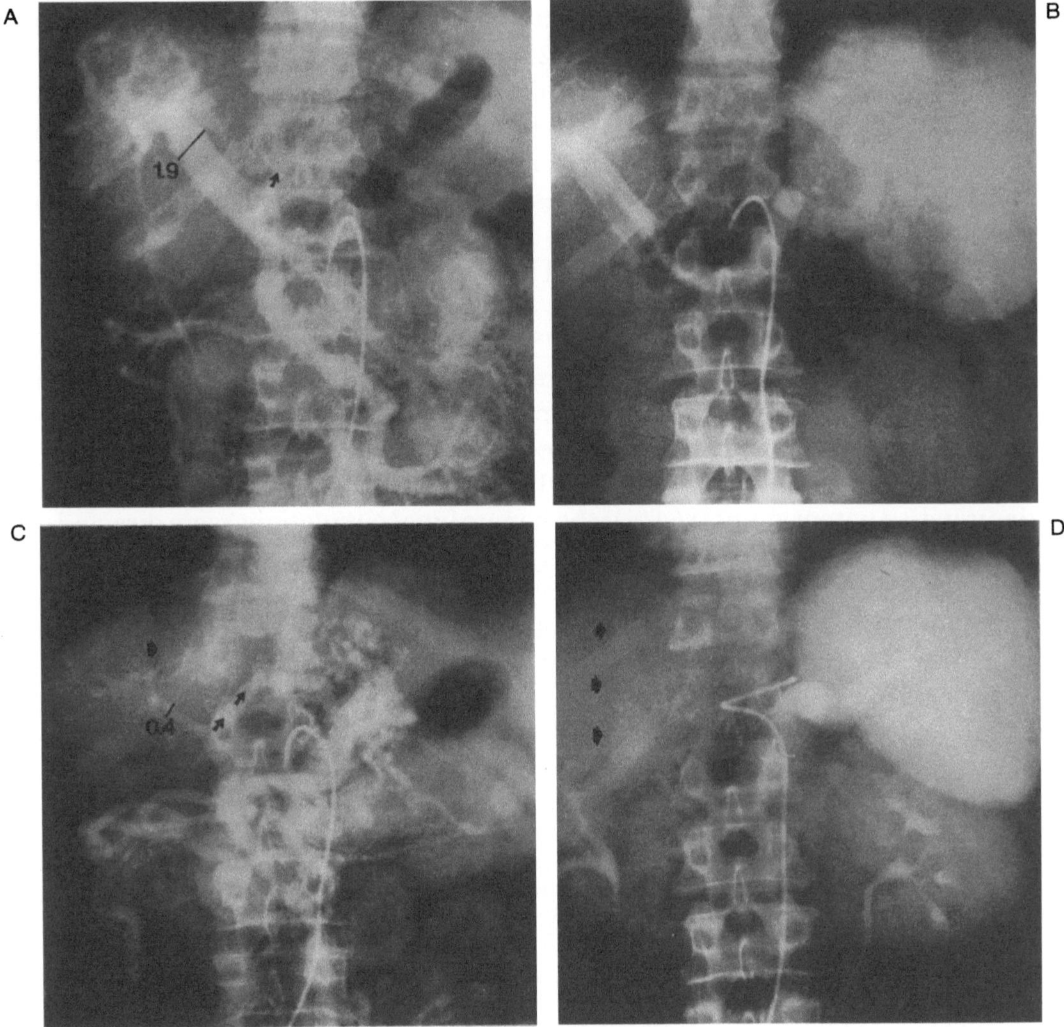

**Fig. 26 A–D.** D. M. (13526/79). Changes in portal circulation.
**A, B** Pre-operative angiography. Portal vein with diameter of 1.9 cm. Retrograde filling of left gastric vein *(arrow,* **A***)*.
**C, D** Postoperative angiography (9 months). **C** In the venous phase of superior mesenteric angiography, very marked reduction in diameter of the portal vein (0.4 cm). The blood flow takes place mainly through the dilated left gastric vein *(arrows),* with good opacification of anastomosis; inferior vena cava is also recognisable *(arrows).*
**D** Confirmation of shunt patency in the venous phase of splenic angiography

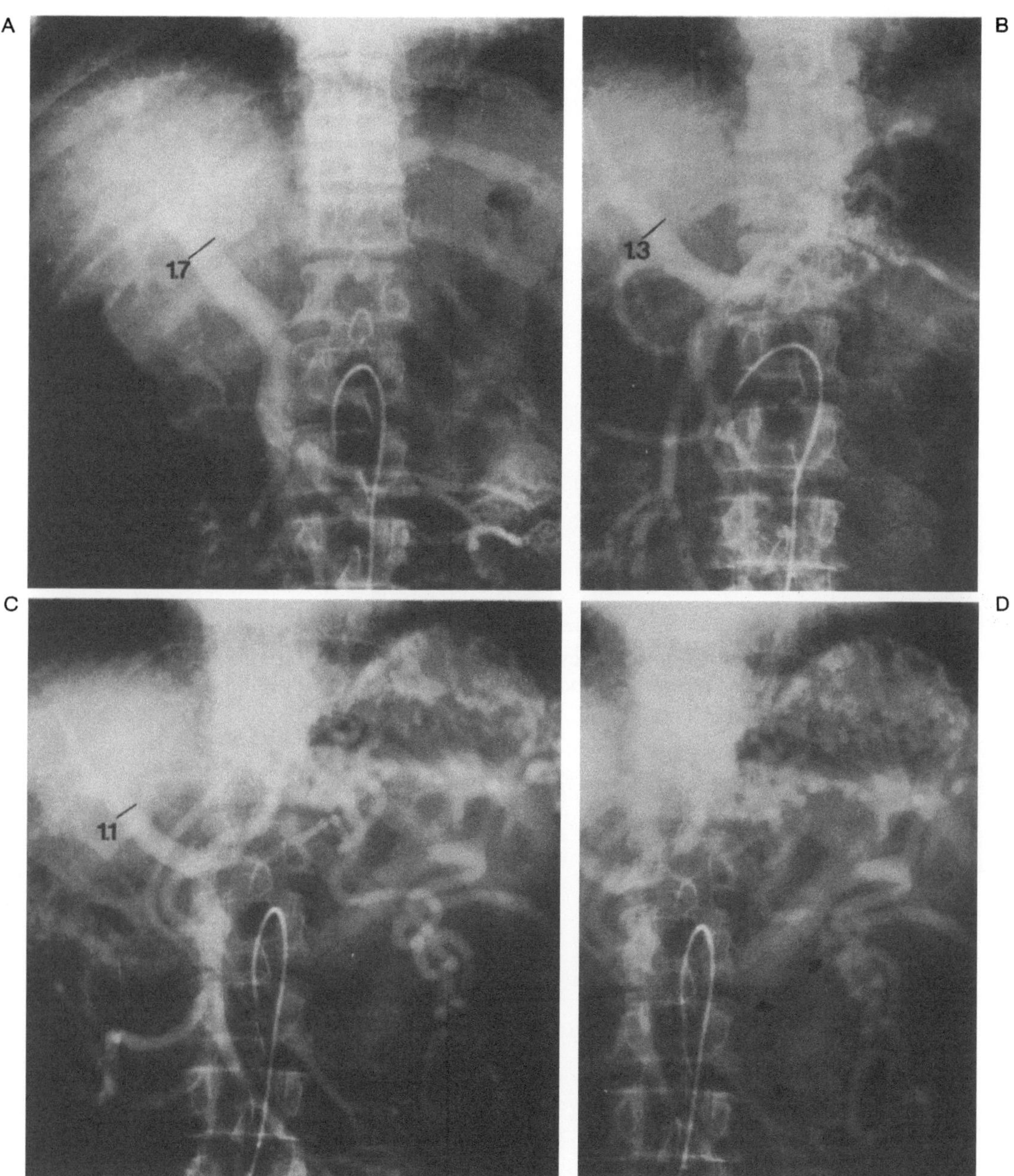

**Fig. 27 A–D.** S. R. (17768/75). Changes in portal circulation. **A** Pre-operative angiography. Portal vein with diameter of 1.7 cm. No hepatofugal circulation is evident. **B** Postoperative angiography: first follow-up (1 month). Reduction in diameter of portal vein (1.3 cm). Development of multiple hepatofugal collaterals directed to large gastric varices. **C, D** Postoperative angiography: second follow-up (16 months). Further reduction in diameter of portal vein (1.1 cm). Hepatofugal collaterals directed to gastric fundus are still evident; development of hepatofugal circulation through mesocolic veins, with opacification of splenic vein and anastomosis *(arrows,* **D***)*

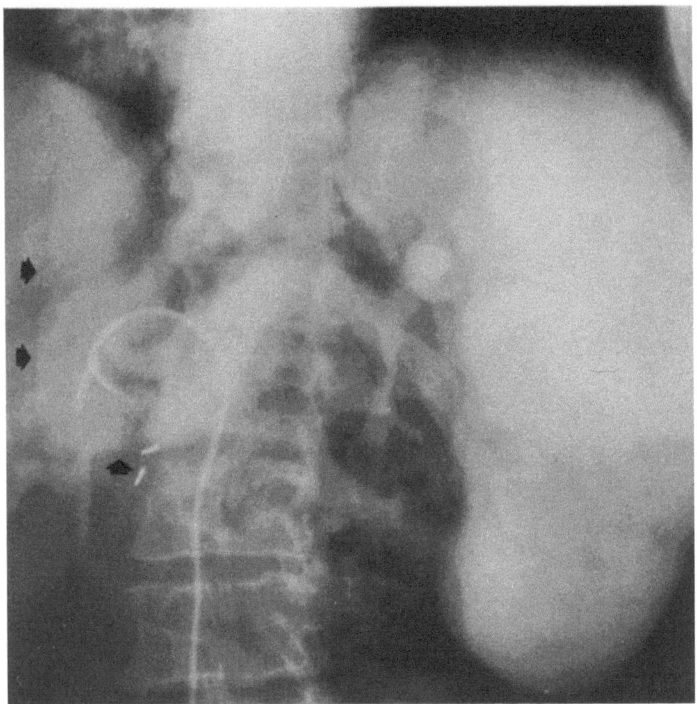

**Fig. 28.** B. A. (10431/76). Shunt patency. Demonstration with arteriography. With selective splenic artery injection, in the venous phase, good opacification of anastomosis, renal vein and inferior vena cava *(arrows)*

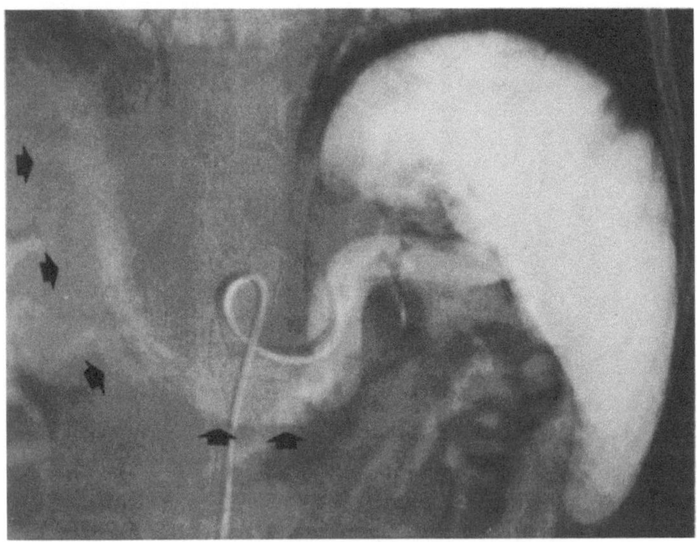

**Fig. 29.** P. F. (14556/77). Shunt patency. Demonstration with arteriography and subtraction. Good opacification of splenic vein. Subtraction allows satisfactory visualization of the renal vein and inferior cava *(arrows)*

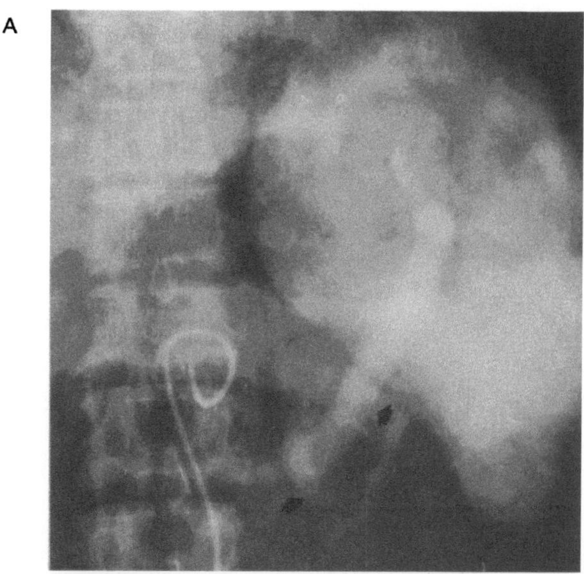

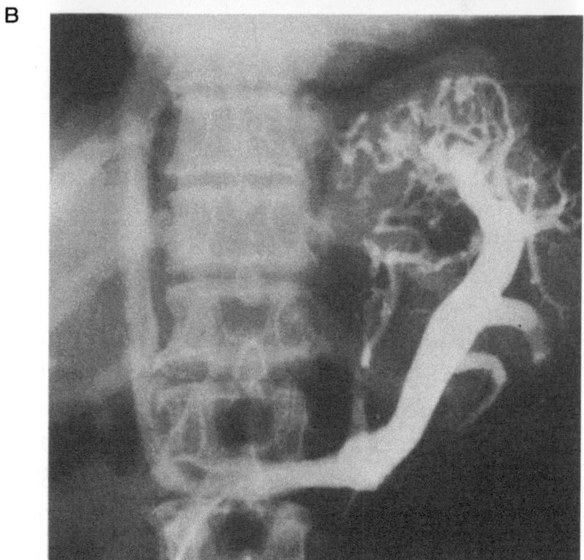

**Fig. 30 A, B.** S. R. (17768/75). Shunt patency. Demonstration with arteriography and shuntography.
**A** In the venous phase of splenic arteriogram, satisfactory visualization of splenic vein as far as anastomosis site *(arrows).* Uncertain visualization of renal vein.
**B** Anastomosography confirms the shunt patency, with good opacification of splenic and renal veins and the inferior vena cava

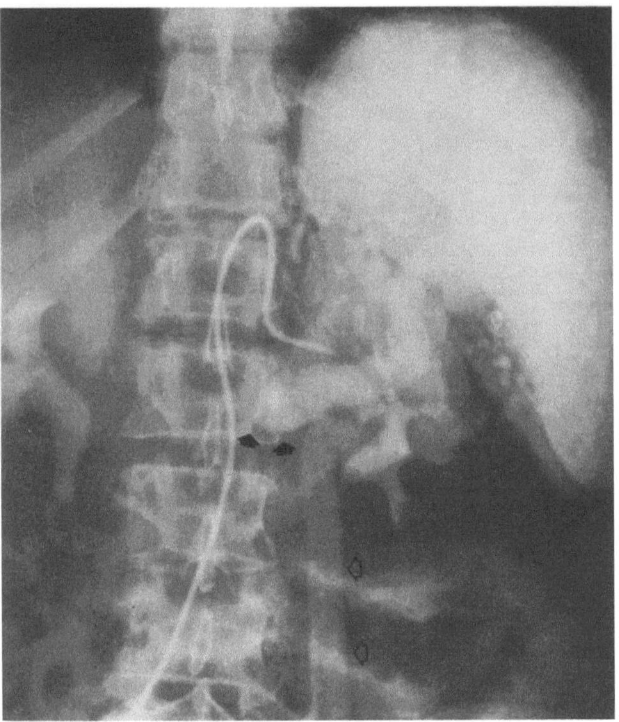

**Fig. 31.** C. E. (1400/77). Shunt patency. Retrograde filling of gonadic vein. Good opacification of splenic vein, anastomosis, and renal vein *(arrows);* feeble opacification of inferior vena cava. Retrograde filling from renal vein of noticeably dilated gonadic vein

cording to NORDLINGER the visualization of the shunt was successful in 54.9% of the cases (he demonstrated patency of the splenic vein in 86%, caval contrast in 81% of cases and renal contrast in 52%. In 7.3% of cases he had to have recourse to direct anastomosography or splenoportography in order to demonstrate the shunt patency. NORDLINGER [59] asserts that – when they occur – distal splenorenal shunt thromboses are early (within 2 weeks), whereas the nonselective shunts tend to occlude more slowly (20 months).

MOSIMANN [53] reports anastomotic thromboses in 9% of cases.

In our set of cases, 23 out of 27 anastomoses (82.5%) were found to be patent with a diagnosis of certainty reached either in the venous phase of arteriography (Figs. 28–31) or through direct anastomosography (Figs. 32, 33). Two shunts with a venous graft and one of the three terminoterminal anastomoses were found to be occluded (Fig. 34).

The effectiveness of the distal splenorenal shunt in terms of effective drainage of the gastro-oesophageal venous bed, also aided by the favourable angle

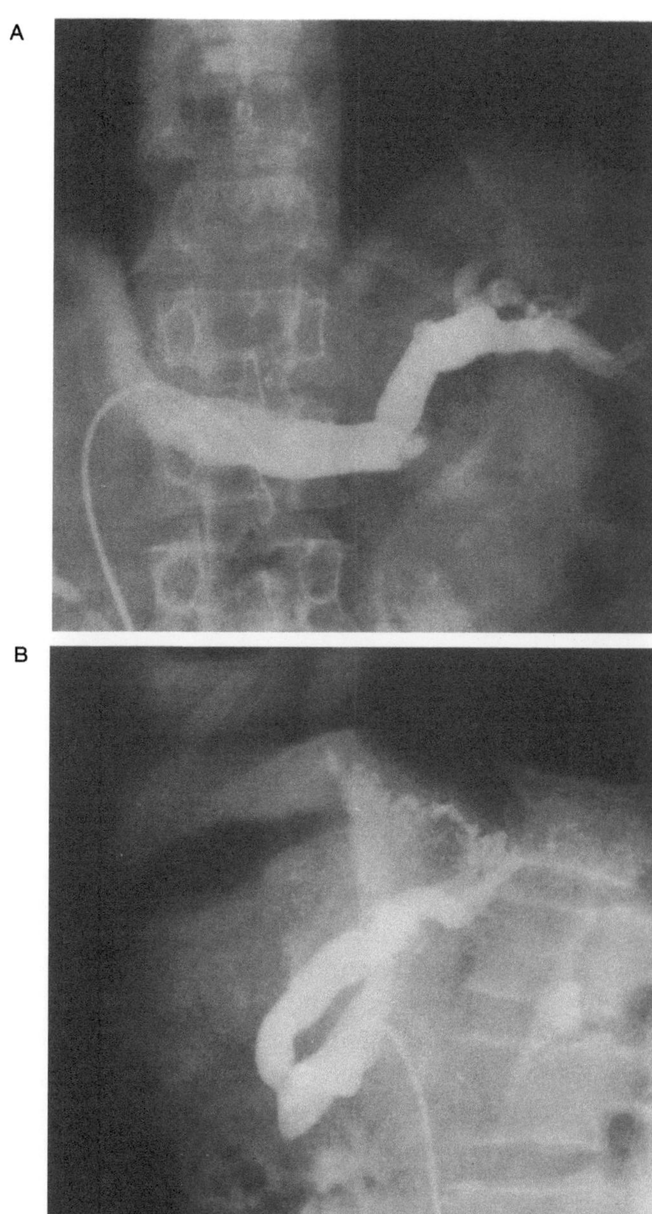

**Fig. 32 A, B.** F. O. (1509/75). Shunt patency. Demonstration with shuntography.
**A** AP projection.
**B** LL projection. Excellent visualization of splenic vein, anastomosis, renal, vein and inferior vena cava. The two orthogonal incidences allow precise evaluation of the calibre of the anastomosis

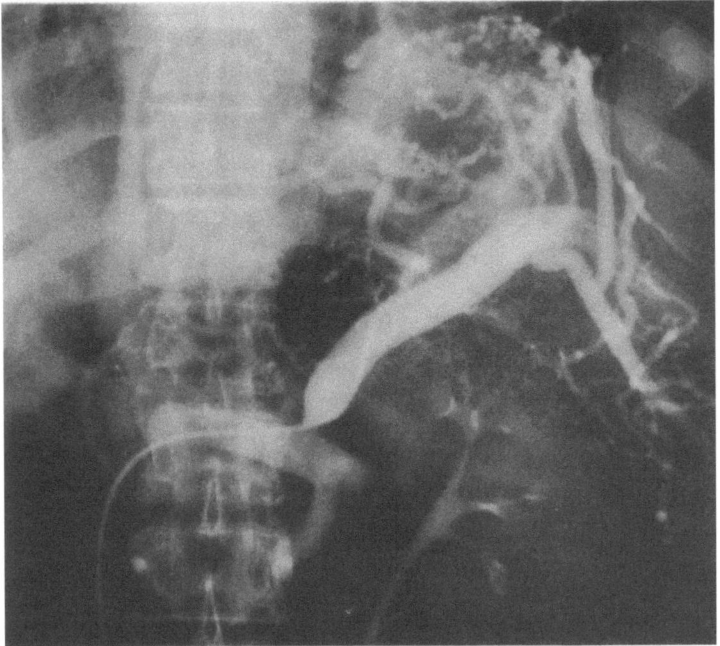

**Fig. 33.** C. E. (1400/77). Shunt patency. Stenosis. Selective catheterization of the splenic vein demonstrates concentric stenosis in anastomosis site

of impact between the splenal vein und the left renal vein [45], is also demonstrated by the *reduction in splenic volume*(Fig. 35) and the *increase in splenic vein diameter,* although without variations affecting the splenic artery (Fig. 36).

BENACERRAF [3] found that the longitudinal axis of the spleen drops from 205 to 179 millimetres. According to SAUBIER [71], the spleen diameter is reduced by 28 mm on average, and according to FUNOVICS [24], a marked reduction in splenic volume is recorded in 59.4% of cases.

NORDLINGER [59] finds a 40% reduction in splenic volume in 88% of cases, and a mean reduction of 31 mm in the spleen's longitudinal axis.

BENACERRAF [3] finds that the splenic vein has increased in diameter at the long-term follow-ups.

In our patients with patent shunts an almost constant decrease in *splenic volume* was observed, with a reduction in longitudinal diameter from a mean of 19 cm (minimum 15, maximum 24) to a mean of 17 cm (minimum 13.5, maximum 24 cm)[3] (Figs. 36, 37, 38). The reduction in splenic volume was observed

---

3  $t = 6.625$, $P < 0.001$, highly significant

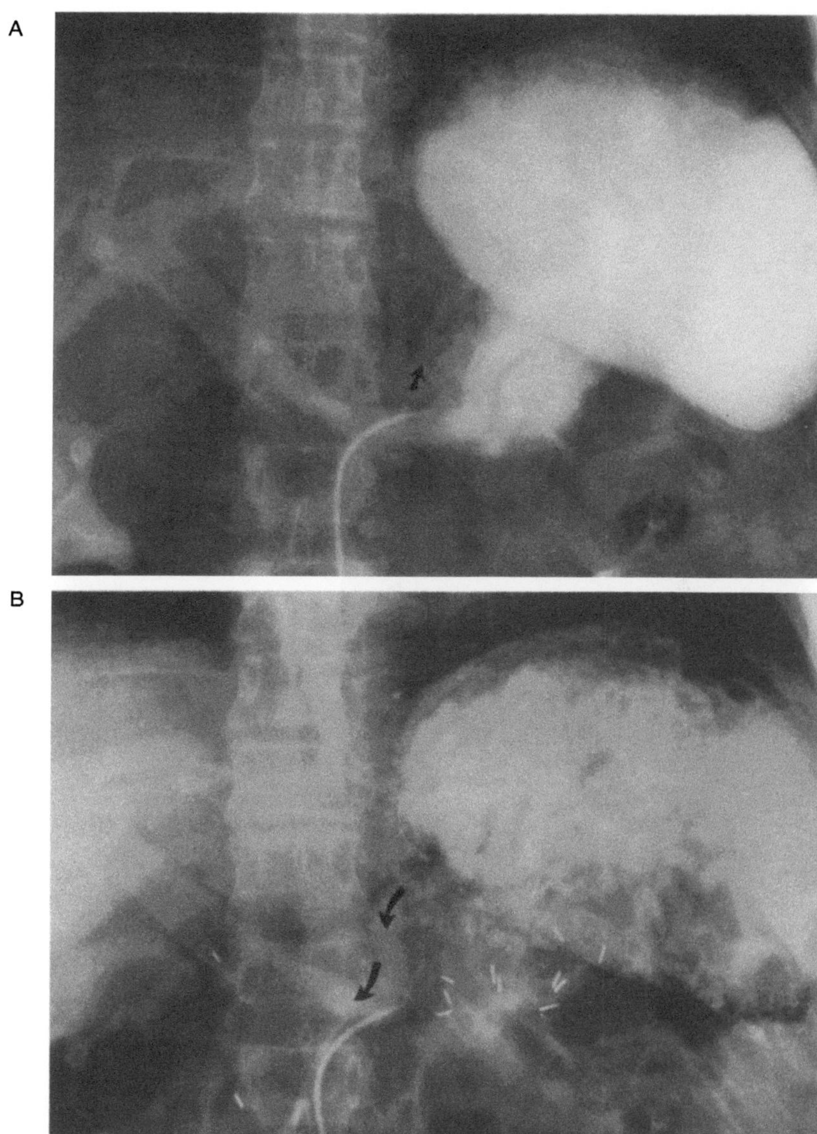

**Fig. 34 A, B.** B. G. (9363/78). Shunt patency. Occlusion.
**A** Pre-operative angiography. Small splenic vein (diameter 1 cm). Hepatofugal flow through left gastric vein *(arrow)*.
**B** Postoperative angiography (1 month). Splenic vein is not opacified. The blood flow takes place through short gastric veins directed to the dilated left gastric vein *(arrows)* and the portal vein

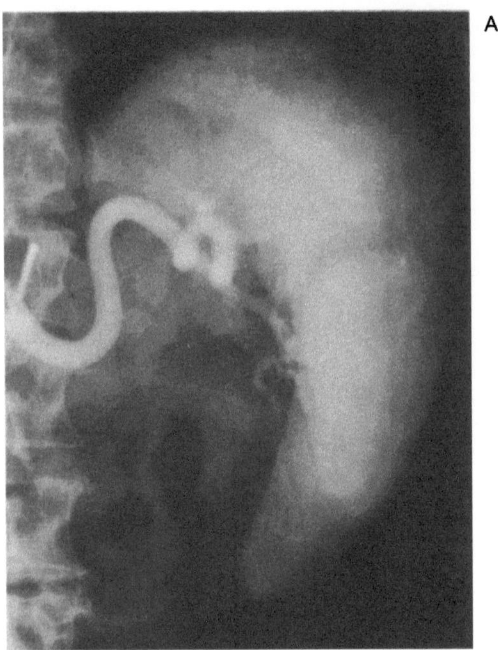

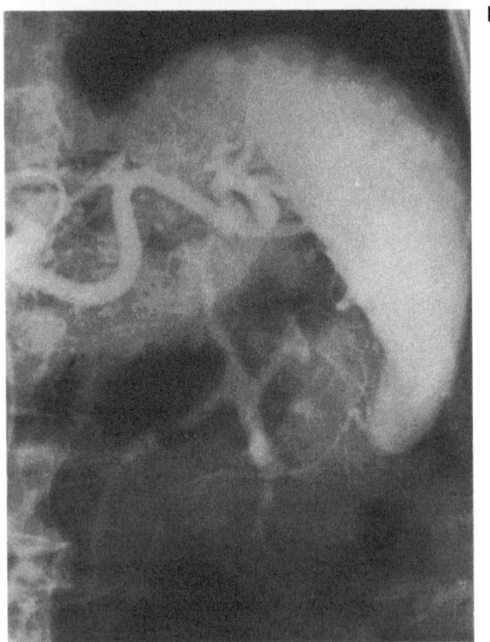

**Fig. 35 A, B.** P. F. (14556/77). Changes in volume of spleen. **A** Pre-operative angiography. Splenic artery with diameter of 0.9 cm. Splenomegaly (longitudinal diameter of spleen 19 cm). **B** Post-operative angiography (28 months). Reduction in diameter of splenic artery (0.7 cm) and in volume of spleen (longitudinal diameter 14.5 cm)

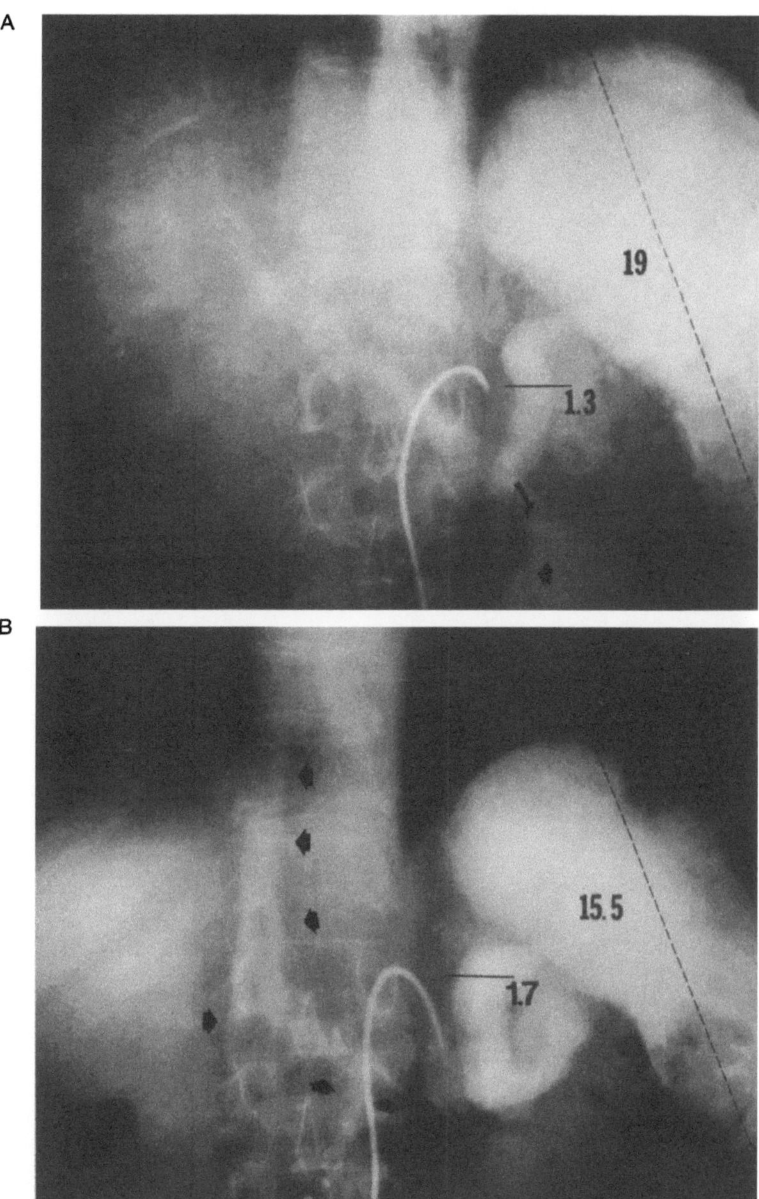

**Fig. 36 A, B.** R. A. (2752/73). Changes of spleen volume and splenic vein diameter.
**A** Pre-operative angiography. Splenomegaly (longitudinal diameter of spleen, 19 cm). Splenic vein with diameter of 1.3 cm. Retrograde filling of inferior mesenteric vein *(arrows)*.
**B** Postoperative angiography (34 months). Noticeable reduction in volume of spleen (longitudinal diameter 15.5 cm). Increase in diameter of splenic vein (1.7 cm). Good evidence of splenorenal shunt patency with opacification of renal vein and inferior vena cava *(arrows)*

Results

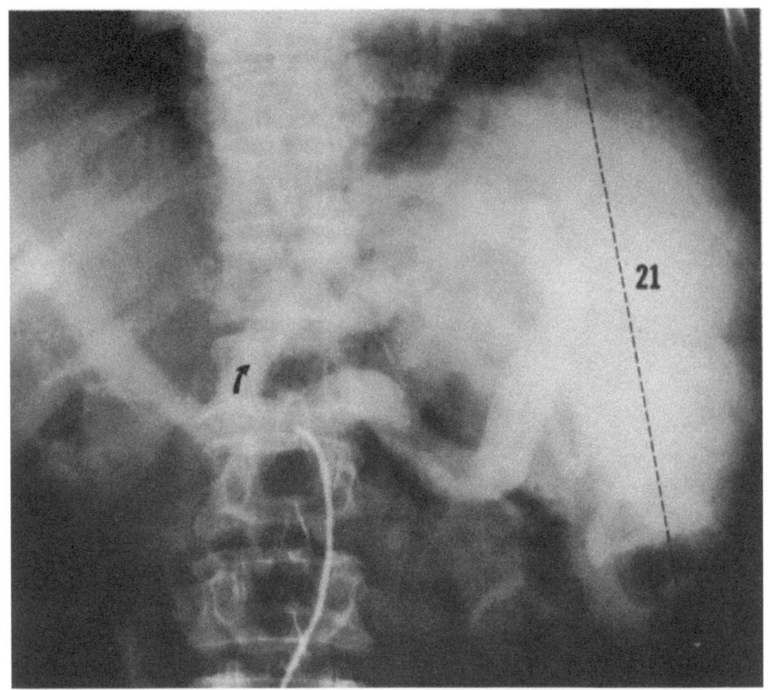

A

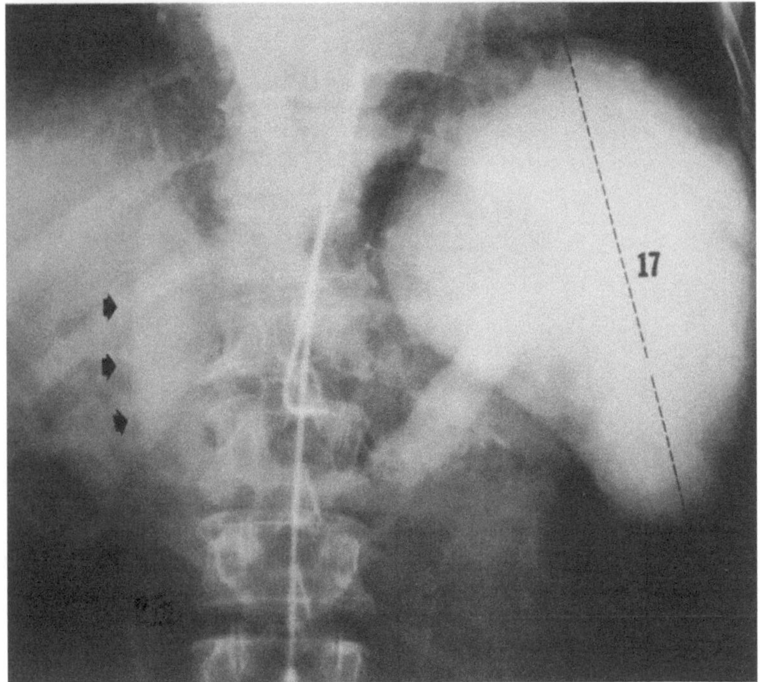

B

60

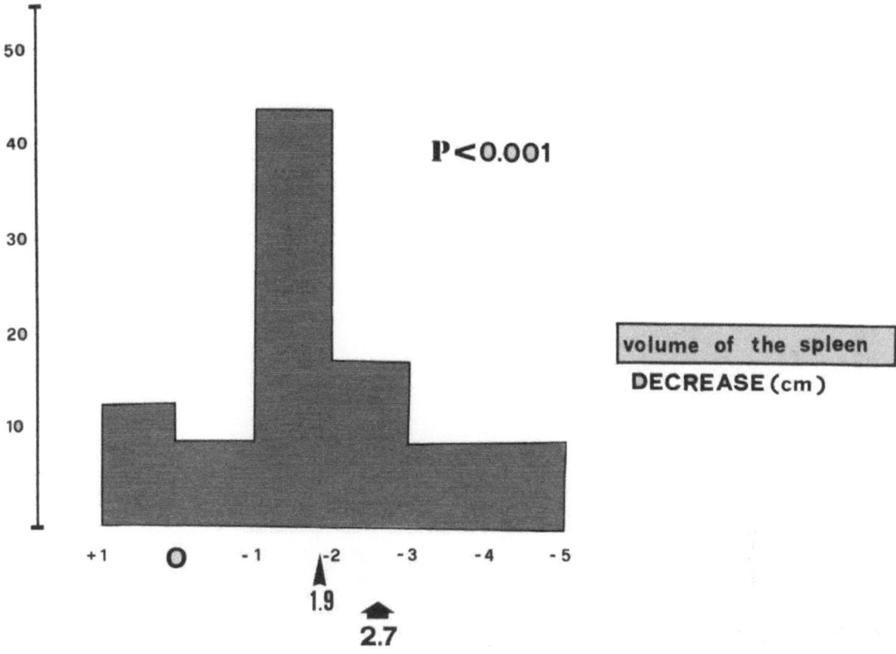


**Fig. 38.** Variations (expressed in centimetres of main longitudinal diameter) in the splenic volume after distal S-R shunt. On the first angiographic control (performed after a mean interval of 6.5 months from the operation) we found *(small arrow)* a mean decrease of 1.9 cm in the longitudinal diameter of the spleen, while on repeated controls (performed after a mean interval of 31 months from the operation) we found a mean decrease of 2.7 cm *(large arrow)*. The postoperative decrease is statistically significant at the 0.001 P level

both in the short-term test and in the long-term follow-ups. Only in two patients with patent shunts was a slight increase in splenic diameter observed (at 2 and 7 months respectively); in a third patient (at 2 months) no changes in volume of the spleen were recorded (Fig. 39). The reduction was progressive in the patients observed a number of times (Fig. 40). Among the patients with occluded shunts, one presented a slight increase in splenic longitudinal diameter.

The *diameter of the splenic artery* did not undergo appreciable variations, even with repeated observations (Fig. 41).

---

**Fig. 37 A, B.** S. R. (17768/75). Changes of spleen volume and splenic vein diameter. **A** Pre-operative angiography. Splenomegaly (longitudinal diameter of spleen, 21 cm). Splenic vein with diameter of 1.8 cm. Hepatofugal flow through left gastric vein *(arrow)*. **B** Postoperative angiography (16 months). Reduction in volume of spleen (longitudinal diameter, 17 cm). No significant change in diameter of splenic vein. Patent shunt with good opacification of inferior vena cava *(arrows)*

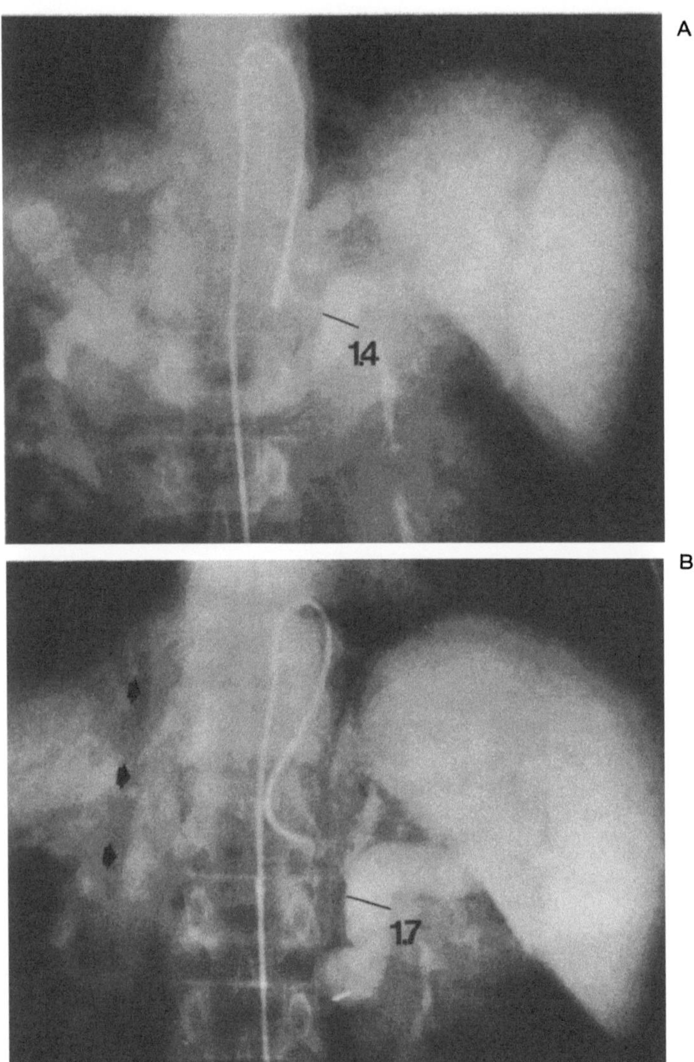

**Fig. 39 A, B.** C. O. (18447/77). Changes of spleen volume and splenic vein diameter.
**A** Pre-operative angiography. Moderate splenomegaly. Splenic vein with diameter of 1.4 cm.
**B** Postoperative angiography (2 months). No significant change in volume of spleen. Increase in diameter of splenic vein (1.7 cm)

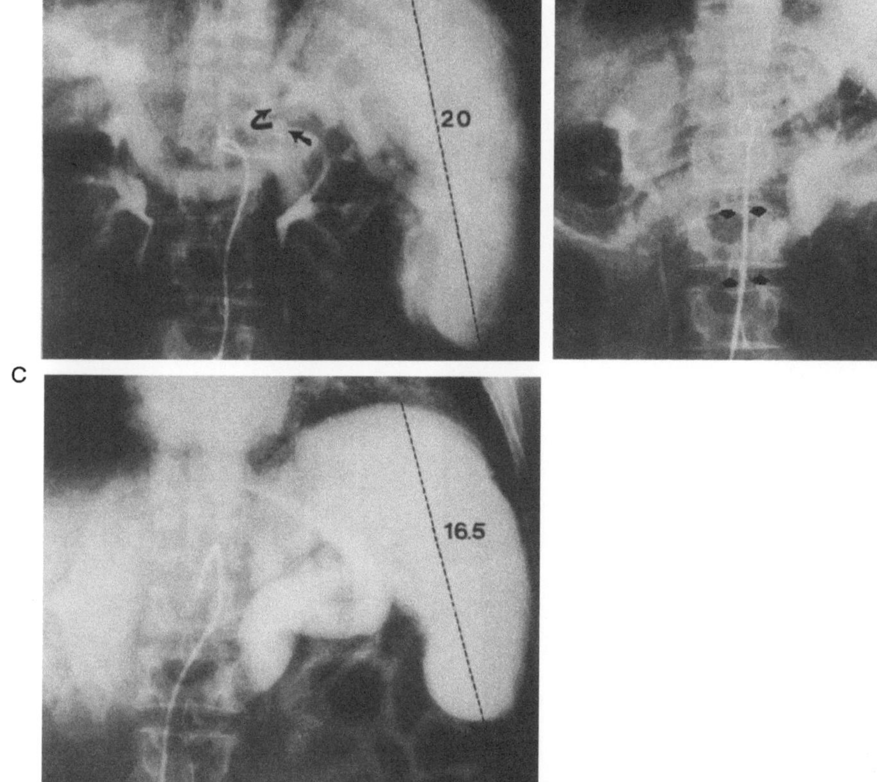

**Fig. 40 A–C.** P. A. (2876/76). Changes of spleen volume and splenic vein diameter. **A** Pre-operative angiography. Splenomegaly (longitudinal diameter of spleen 20 cm). Splenic vein with diameter of 1.5 cm. Hepatofugal flow through dilated short gastric veins *(arrows)*. **B** Postoperative angiography. First follow-up (1 month). Slight reduction in volume of spleen (longitudinal diameter of 18.5 cm). Splenic vein with unchanged diameter. Patent anastomosis; feeble opacification of renal vein *(arrows)*. **C** Postoperative angiography: second follow-up (49 months). Further reduction in volume of spleen (longitudinal diameter of 16.5 cm); increase in diameter of splenic vein (1.9 cm). Much better demonstration of shunt patency with good opacification of renal vein and inferior vena cava

Among the 23 patients with permeable shunts, 17 presented an increase in *splenic vein diameter* from a mean of 1.30 cm (minimum 0.9, maximum 1.8) to a mean of 1.6 cm (minimum 0.9, maximum 2.2)[4] (Figs. 42, 43). The increase in splenic vein diameter was progressive in the repeated tests.

---

4 $t = 5.331$, $P < 0.001$, highly significant

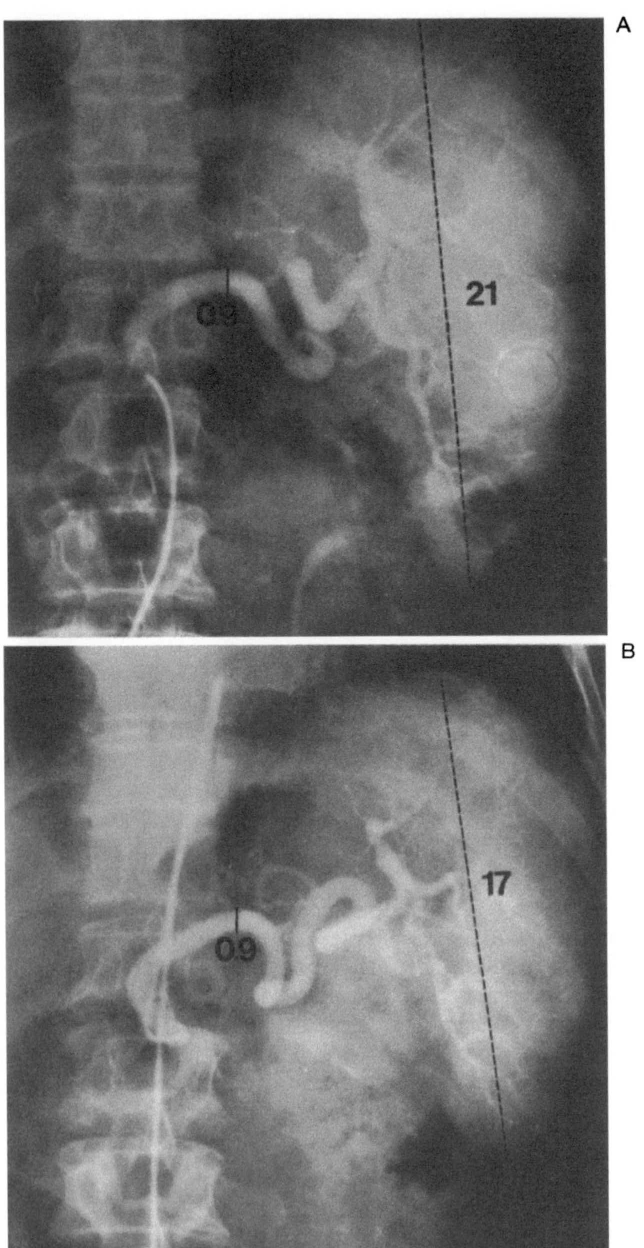

**Fig. 41 A, B.** S. R. (17768/75). Changes in diameter of splenic artery.
**A** Pre-operative angiography. Splenic artery with diameter 0.9 cm. Splenomegaly (longitudinal diameter of spleen, 21 cm).
**B** Postoperative angiography (16 months). Splenic artery with diameter unchanged. Noticeable reduction in volume of spleen (longitudinal diameter, 17 cm)

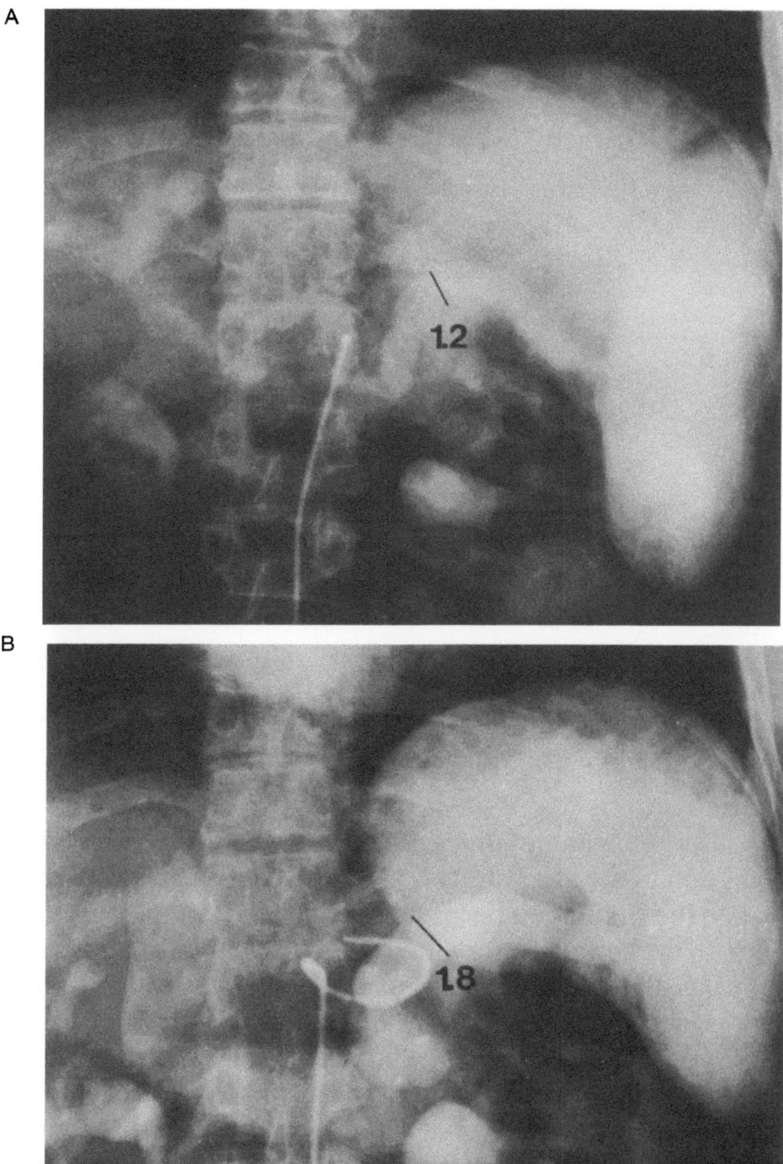



**Fig. 42 A, B.** M. G. (799/78). Changes of spleen volume and splenic vein diameter.
**A** Pre-operative angiography. Splenomegaly (longitudinal diameter of spleen, 19 cm). Splenic vein with diameter of 1.2 cm. **B** Postoperative angiography (27 months). Reduction in volume of spleen (longitudinal diameter, 16.5 cm). Increased diameter of splenic vein (1.8 cm). The anastomosis is patent with noticeable dilatation of renal vein

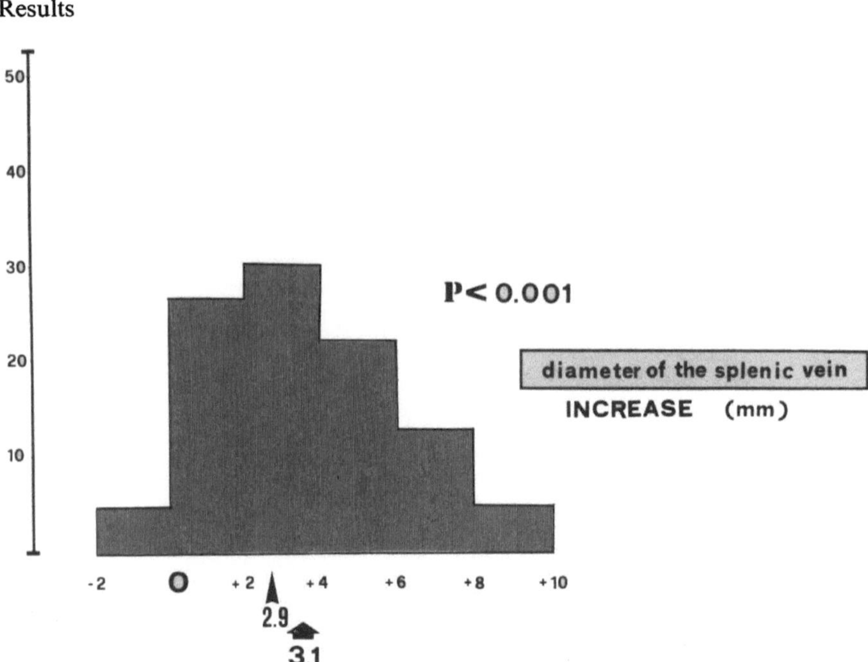



**Fig. 43.** Variations (expressed in millimetres) in the diameter of the splenic vein after distal S-R shunt. On the first angiographic control (performed after a mean interval of 6.5 months from the operation) we found a mean increase of 2.9 mm *(small arrow),* while on repeated controls (performed after a mean interval of 31 months from the operation) we found a mean increase of 3.1 mm *(large arrow).* The postoperative increase is statistically significant at the 0.001 P level

The behaviour of the *hepatic artery diameter* (Fig. 44) is variously commented upon in the literature. NABSETH [57] states that in the long-term follow-ups, when the circulation becomes hepatofugal but there is no encephalopathy, it is due to the compensatory increased capacity of the arterial flow. According to WIDRICH [94], the diameter of the hepatic artery in two cases he studied increased from 0.8 to 0.95 cm at 23 months, and from 0.5 to 1 cm at 26 months.

NORDLINGER [59], on the contrary, did not observe hepatic artery diameter changes – in agreement with BENACERRAF [3] – in either the early or late tests.

In our cases the *volume of the liver* is appreciably reduced; the mean longitudinal diameter dropped from 19.87 cm (minimum 13, maximum 27) to 17.41 cm (minimum 11, maximum 25.5). The reduction in hepatic volume was progressive. Only in 2 out of 23 patients (examined at 28 and 45 months) was no reduction found.

In 7 of the 21 patients with reduction of the hepatic volume there was an associated increase in the tortuousness of the intrahepatic arterial branches.

The *hepatic artery diameter* increased from a mean of 0.64 cm to a mean of 0.69 cm (Figs. 45, 46).

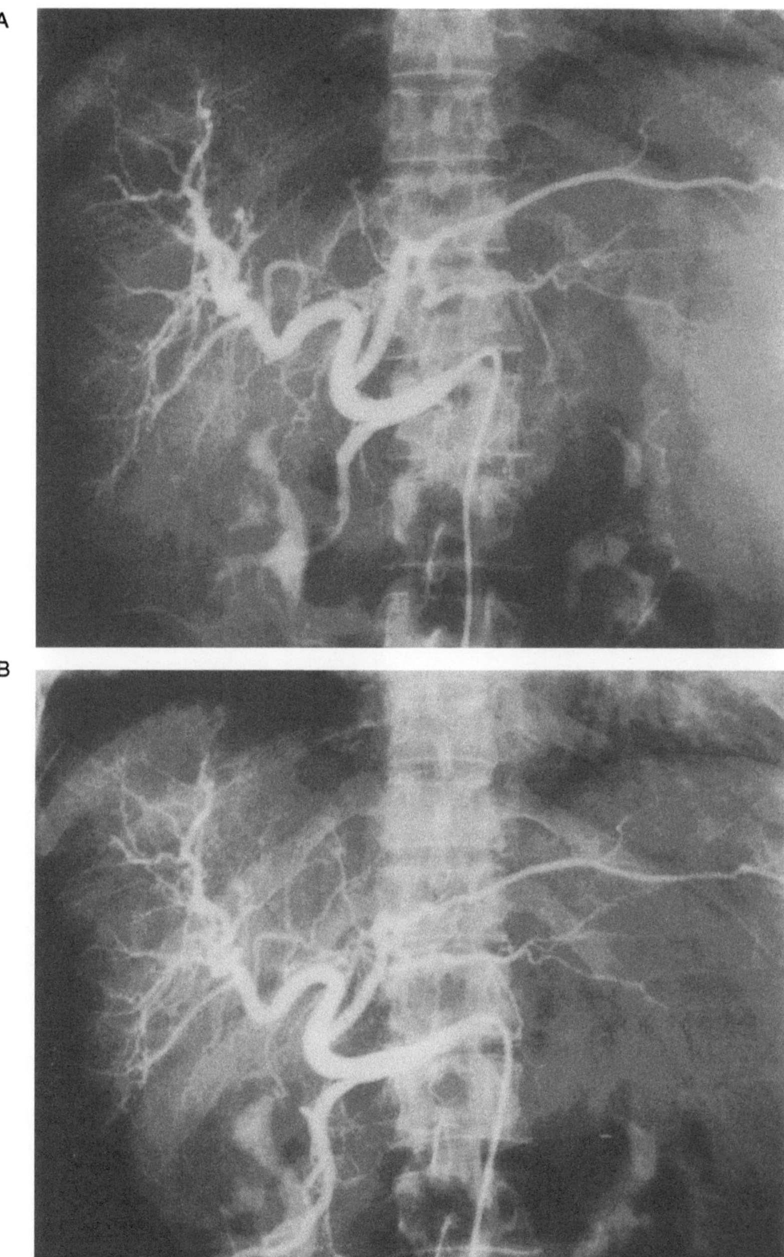

**Fig. 44 A, B.** L. M. (973/80). Changes in diameter of hepatic artery and course of intrahepatic branches. **A** Pre-operative angiography. Hepatic artery of good diameter. Branches for right lobe moderately tortuous; branches for left lobe stretched (hypertrophy of left lobe). **B** Postoperative angiography (5 months). No significant changes of the picture

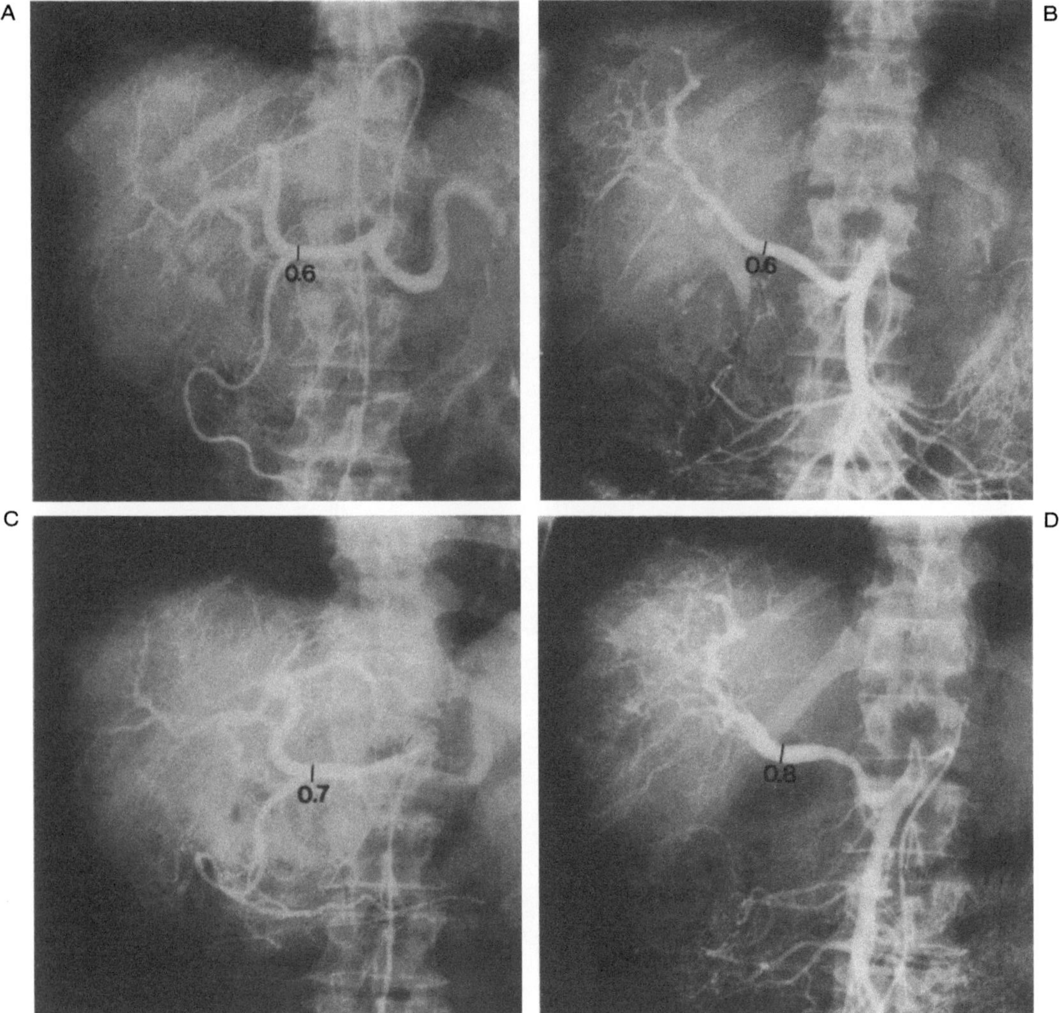

**Fig. 45 A–D.** P. F. (14556/77). Changes in diameter of hepatic artery and course of intrahepatic branches.

**A, B** Pre-operative angiography. Presence of accessory right hepatic artery originating from superior mesenteric artery. Both hepatic arteries have good diameter (0.6 cm) with moderately tortuous branches, especially those directed to right lobe.

**C, D** Postoperative angiography (28 months). Increase in diameter of hepatic arteries originating from coeliac trunk (0.7 cm) and superior mesenteric artery (0.8 cm). Intrahepatic branches more tortuous, especially in right lobe, which is considerably reduced in volume (the reduction in diameter at proximal tract of right accessory hepatic artery may be attributed to a previous attempt at selective catheterization)

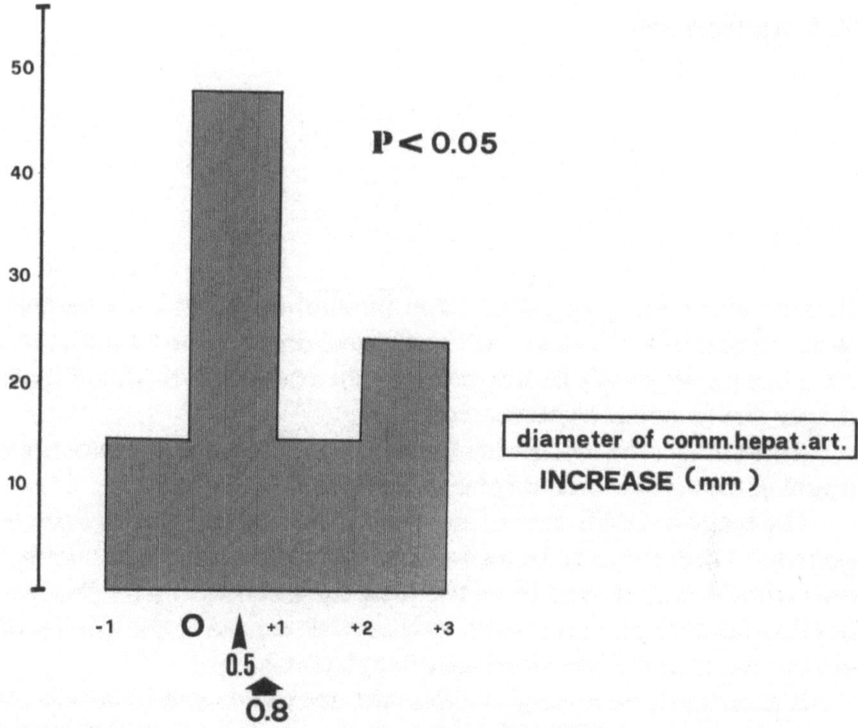


**Fig. 46.** The diagram shows the variations (expressed in millimeters) in the diameter of the common hepatic artery, after distal S-R shunt. On the first angiographic control (performed after a mean interval of 6.5 months from the operation) we found *(small arrow)* a mean increase of 0.5 mm, while on repeated controls (performed after a mean interval of 31 months from the operation) we found *(large arrow)* a mean increase of 0.8 mm.
The postoperative increase is statistically significant at the 0.05 P level

# 9. Conclusions

In light of the foregoing data from the literature, the conclusions must inevitably consist in a question: do the clinical and haemodynamic results of Warren's operation justify its adoption as the operation of first choice in haemorrhages due to portal hypertension?

Apart from schistosomiasis (a case in which there does not appear to be any doubts), the answer can only be subjective.

The technical difficulty of the operation's performance does not – with experience – seem to us to be an unsurmountable obstacle, while the fact that the operation is not, at least from the long-term standpoint, selective clearly does not invalidate the better results, at least with regard to the quality of life and the effectiveness of the haemorrhagic prophylaxis.

It is certainly necessary to assess the operation and its results even more extensively; we nevertheless feel that at present it constitutes the best available approximation within the field of treatment of the haemorrhagic symptom of cirrhosis of the liver [50, 51].

# 10. References


1. ABEATICI S, DORIGO M, GHIGO M, JIULIANI G (1979) Correlazioni tra reperti splenoportografici e rischio di emorragie digestive nell'ipertensione portale. Minerva Chir 34: 453
2. BAKER LA, SMITH C, LIEBERMANN G (1959) The natural history of esophageal varices. Am J Med 2: 228
3. BENACERRAF R, VERMELIN P, DANIEL B (1979) L'anastomose splenorenale distale de Warren. J Radiol 60: 493
4. BENGMARK S (1975) Surgical management of portal hypertension. Clin Gastroenterol 4: 395
5. BERCHTOLD R (1976) Der Warren-Shunt. Langenbecks Arch Chir 342: 153
6. BERCHTOLD R (1978) Soll man Patienten mit portaler Hypertension operieren? Schweiz Med Wochenschr 108: 1046
7. BISMUTH H, FRANCO D (1976) Portal diversion for portal hypertension in early childhood. Ann Surg 183: 439
8. BRITTON RC (1977) The clinical effectiveness of selective portal shunts. Am J Surg 133: 506
9. BURCHARTH F, NIELBO N, ANDERSEN B (1979) Percutaneous transhepatic portography. Comparison with splenoportography in portal hypertension. Am J Roentgenol 132: 183
10. BURCHELL AR, MORENO AH, PANKE WF, NEALON TF (1976) Hepatic artery flow improvement after p-c shunt: a single haemodynamic clinical correlate. Ann Surg 184: 289
11. BUSUTTIL RW, BRIN B, TOMPKINS RK (1979) Matched control study of distal splenorenal and portacaval shunts in the treatment of bleeding esophageal varices. Am J Surg 138: 62
12. CAMPBELL DP, PARKER DE, ANAGNOSTOPOULOS CE (1973) Survival prediction in portacaval shunts: a computerized statistical analysis. Am J Surg 126: 748
13. CARLSON RE, EHRENFELD WK (1976) Recurrent variceal hemorrhage following successful Warren shunt. Arch Surg 111: 587
14. CONN HO, RAMSBY GR (1973) Angiographic techniques in assessing the patency of portacaval anastomoses. Dig Dis 18: 651
15. CONN HO, LIEBERTHAL MM (1979) The hepatic coma syndromes. Williams & Wilkins, Baltimore
16. COOPERMAN AM, HERMANN RE (1977) Ligation procedures in the management of portal hypertension. Surgery 81: 382
17. DAGRADI AE, STEMPIEN SJ, TAN DT (1970) Endoscopic study of the cirrhotic patient before and following portacaval shunt for bleeding varices. Am J Gastroenterol 55: 425
18. Del GUERCIO LRM, COHN JD, KAZARIAN KK, KINKHABWALLA M (1978) A shunt equation for estimating the splenic component of portal hypertension. Am J Surg 135: 70
19. ECKHAUSER FE, STRODEL WE, TURCOTTE JG (1980) Hemodynamics in portal hypertension. In: Fiddian-Green RG, Turcotte JG (eds) Gastrointestinal Hemorrhage. Grune & Stratton, New York, p 235
20. FELIX WR, MYERSON RM, SIGEL B, PERRIN EB, JACKSON FC (1974) The effect of portacaval shunt on hypersplenism. Surg Gynecol Obstet 139: 899
21. FERRARA J, ELLISON EC, MARTIN EW, COOPERMAN M (1979) Correction of hypersplenism following distal splenorenal shunt. Surgery 86: 570

References

22. Frasson F, Fugazzola C, Di Palma A, Marzoli GP (1977) Bilancio angiografico nell'ipertensione portale, In: La Radiologia dell' esofago, dello stomaco e del duodeno. Arti Grafiche Bertoncello, Cittadella (PD)
23. Fulenwider JT, Nordlinger BM, Millikan WJ, Sones PJ, Warren WD (1979) Portal pseudoperfusion. Ann Surg 189: 257
24. Funovics J, Mülbacher F, Fritsch A, Appel WH (1979) Preliminary results with the distal splenorenal shunt. Langenbecks Arch Chir 349: 576
25. Funovics J, Fritsch A, Mühlbacher F, Appel W (1979) Hämodynamik, Enzephalopathie und Lebensqualität nach distalem splenorenalem Shunt (Warren-Shunt). Acta Chir Austriaca 25: 509
26. Galambos JT, Rudman D, Warren WD (1976) Portal hypertension, a new beginning for an old problem. Dig Dis 21: 827
27. Garceau AJ, Chalmers TC (1963) The natural history of cirrhosis. N Engl J Med 268: 469
28. Göthlin J, Tylen U (1976) Blood flow determination in splenorenal shunts using a dye dilution technique. Acta Chir Scand 142: 155
29. Grauer SE, Schwartz SI (1979) Extrahepatic portal hypertension: a retrospective analysis. Ann Surg 189: 566
30. Guharay BN, Sain P, Sengupta KP, Mallick KK, Biswas S, Basu AK (1978) Graft interposition splenocaval shunt for total or selective decompression of portal hypertension. Surgery 83: 164
31. Gutgemann A, Esser G, Cerny J, Schulz D (1970) Klinische Erfahrungen zum Pfortaderhochdruck. Bruns' Beitr Klin Chir 218: 97
32. Henley KS, Clifford LH, Nostrant TT (1980) Gastrointestinal hemorrage, portacaval shunts and hepatic reserve. In: Fiddian-Green RG, Turcotte JG (eds) Gastrointestinal Hemorrhage. Grune & Stratton, New York, p 253
33. Hutson DG, Pereiras R, Zeppa R, Levi JU, Schiff ER, Fink P (1976) The fate of esophageal varices following selective distal splenorenal shunt. Ann Surg 183: 496
34. Hutson DG, Zeppa R, Levi JU, Schiff ER, Livingstone AS, Fink P (1977) The effect of the distal splenorenal shunt on hypersplenism. Ann Surg 185: 605
35. James EC, Fedde CW, Khuri NT, Gillespie JT (1978) Division of the left renal vein: a safe surgical adjunct. Surgery 83: 151
36. Johansson B (1976) Structural and functional changes in rat portal vein after experimental portal hypertension. Acta Physiol Scand 98: 381
37. Kessler RE, Tice DA, Zimmon DS (1969) Retrograde flow of portal vein blood in patients with cirrhosis. Radiology 92: 1038
38. Langer B, Rotstein LE, Stone RM, Taylor BR, Patel SC, Blendis LM, Colapinto RF (1980) A prospective selective trial of the selective distal spleno-renal shunt. Surg Gynecol Obstet 150: 45
39. Law DK, Moore EE (1979) Compartmentalized gastrosplenic and mesenteric venous hypertension after distal splenorenal shunt occlusion: response to mesocaval shunt and splenectomy. Surgery 85: 579
40. Le Cudonnec B, Bigot JM (1976) La phlebographie sus-hepatique. Ann Radiol (Paris) 19: 405
41. Leger L (1978) Hemorragies digestives de l'hypertension portale. Nouv Presse Med 27: 2363
42. Lemaigre G, Louvel A, Achour H (1978) Hemorragies digestives de l'hypertension portale. Nouv Presse Med 27: 2367
43. Levi JU, Zeppa R, Hutson DG, Civetta JM, Ono J, Smith JP, Etlimg T (1976) Early hemodynamic effects of the distal splenorenal shunt. Surg Forum 27: 370
44. Loup P, Mosimann R (1977) Repercussion spleniques du shunt spleno-renal distal selon Warren. Helv Chir Acta 44: 477

45. Maillard JN, Flamant YM, Hay JM, Chandler JG (1979) Selectivity of the distal spleno-renal shunt. Surgery 86: 663

46. Maksoud JG, Miles S, Pinto VC (1978) Distal-splenorenal shunt in children. J Pediatr Surg 13: 335

47. Malt RA (1976) Portasystemic venous shunts (two parts). N Engl J Med 295: 24/80

48. Malt RA, Nabseth DC, Orloff MJ, Stipa S (1979) Portal hypertension, 1979. N Engl J Med 301: 617

49. Martin EW, Molnar J, Coopermann M, Pace WG, Thomford NR, Carey LC (1978) Observations on fifty distal splenorenal shunts. Surgery 84: 379

50. Marzoli GP, Vesentini S, Frasson F, Fugazzola C, Mangiante G (1979) Die distale spleno-renale termino-laterale Anastomose nach Warren. Langenbecks Arch Chir 348: 93

51. Marzoli GP, Vesentini S, Mangiante G, Frasson F, Fugazzola C, Tenchini P (1979) Klinische und hämodynamische Evaluation der distalen selektiven spleno-renalen Anastomose nach Warren. Helv Chir Acta 46: 807

52. Mathie RT, Toouli J, Smith A, Harper AM, Blumgart LH (1980) Hepatic tissue perfusion studies during distal splenorenal shunt. Am J Surg 140: 384

53. Mosimann R, Loup P (1977) Efficacy and risks of the distal splenorenal shunt in the treatment of bleeding esophageal varices. Am J Surg 133: 163

54. Mülbacher F, Funovics J, Rauhs R, Fritsch A (1979) Hämodinamik der portalen Hypertension-Mythos oder Realität. Langenbecks Arch Chir 349: 575

55. Mutchnick MG, Lerner E, Conn HO (1974) Portal-systemic encephalopathy and portacaval anastomosis: a prospective, controlled investigation. Gastroenterology 66: 1005

56. Nabseth DC, Widrich WC, O'Hara ET, Johnson WC (1975) Flow and pressure characteristics of the portal system before and after splenorenal shunts. Surgery 78: 739

57. Nabseth DC, Johnson WC, Widrich WC, O'Hara ET, Vollman RW (1979) Splenorenal shunts in portal hypertension. J Cardiovasc Surg (Torino) 20: 201

58. Nordlinger BM, Fulenwider JT, Millikan WJ, Warren WD (1978) Splenic artery ligation in distal splenorenal shunts. Am J Surg 136: 561

59. Nordlinger BM, Nordlinger DF, Fulenwider JT, Millikan WJ, Sones PJ, Kutner M, Steete R, Bain R, Warren WD (1980) Angiography in portal hypertension. Am J Surg 139: 132

60. Peto R, Pike MC, Armitage P, Breslow NE, Cox DR, Howard SV, Mantel N, Mc Pherson K, Peto J, Smith PC (1976) Design and analysis of randomized clinical trials requiring prolonged observation of each patient. Br J Cancer 34: 585

61. Pezzuoli G, Spina GP (1978) I problemi clinici dell'ipertensione portale. Minerva Chir 33: 977

62. Powell WJ, Klatskin G (1968) Duration of survival in patients with Laennec's cirrhosis. Am J Med 44: 406

63. Puttini M, Marni A, Montes F, Belli L (1979) Effect of portasystemic shunt on hypersplenism: clinical study in 129 patients with cirrhosis. Am Surg 45: 444

64. Reichle FA (1972) Portal hemodynamics after distal splenorenal shunt. Ann Surg 176: 195

65. Reichle FA, Fahmy WF, Golsorkhi M (1979) Prospective comparative clinical trial with distal splenorenal and mesocaval shunts. Am J Surg 137: 13

66. Resnick RH, Atterbury CE, Grace ND, Conn HO (1979) Distal splenorenal shunt vs. portalsystemic shunt: current status of a controlled trial (Abstr). Gastroenterol: 77 No 5

67. Rikkers LF, Rudman D, Galambos JT, Fulenwider JT, Millikan WJ, Kutner M, Smith RB, Salam AF, Jones PJ, Warren WD (1978) A randomized, controlled trial of the distal splenorenal shunt. Ann Surg 188: 271

68. Rodgers BM, Talbert JL (1979) Distal splenorenal shunt for portal decompression in childhood. J Pediatr Surg 14: 33

References

69. ROTSTEIN LE, MAKOWKA L, LANGER B, BLENDIS LM, STONE RM, COLAPINTO RF (1979) Thrombosis of the portal vein following distal splenorenal shunt. Surg Gynecol Obstet 149: 847
70. SATIANI B, LIAPIS C, EVANS WE (1980) Kinking of a Warren shunt as a cause of recurrent variceal hemorrage. Am J Surg 139: 428
71. SAUBIER EC, PARTENSKY C, PINET A, LYONNET D, GOUILLAT C (1980) Operation de Warren pour hypertension portale, appreciation de la methode par controle angiographique precoce de 23 cas. J Chir (Paris) 117: 147
72. SHERLOCK S (1978) Portal circulation and portal hypertension. Gut 19: 70
73. SIEGEL JH, GOLDWYN RM, FARRELL EJ, GALLIN P, FRIEDMAN HP (1974) Hyperdynamic states and the physiologic determinants of survival. Arch Surg 108: 282
74. SILVER D, PUCKETT CL, MCNEER JF, MCLEOD ME, SABINSTON DC (1974) Evaluation of selective transsplenic decompression of gastroesophageal varices. Am J Surg 127: 30
75. SIMERT G, LUNDERQUIST A, TYLEN U, VANG J (1978) Correlatio between percutaneous transhepatic portography and clinical findings in 56 patients with portal hypertension. Acta Chir Scand 144: 27
76. SIMERT G, PERSSON T, VANG J (1978) Factors predicting survival after portacaval shunt. Ann Surg 187: 174
77. SMITH GW (1979) The distal splenorenal shunt (Editorial) Surgery 86: 774
78. SMITH-LAING G, CAMILO ME, DICK R, SHERLOCK S (1980) Percutaneous transhepatic portography in the assessment of portal hypertension. Gastroenterology 78: 197
79. SONES PJ, RUDE JC, BERG DJ, WARREN WD (1978) Evaluation of the left renal vein in candidates for splenorenal shunts. Diagn Radiol 127: 357
80. STARZL TE, PORTER KA, KASHIWAGI N, LEE IY, RUSSELL WJI, PUTNAM CW (1975) The effect of diabetes mellitus on portal blood hepatotrophic factors in dogs. Surg Gynecol Obstet 140: 549
81. SWAN KG, SWAN RC (1980) Some anatomical considerations relevant to the creation of selective splenorenal shunts. Am Surg 46: 298
82. THOMFORD NR (1975) Abnormal left renal vein. Am J Surg 129: 503
83. THOMFORD NR, SIRINEK KR, MARTIN EW (1975) A series of 20 successful Warren shunts. Arch Surg 110: 584
84. TYLEN U, SIMERT G, VANG J (1976) Hemodynamic changes after distal splenorenal shunt studied by sequential angiography. Diagn Radiol 121: 585
85. VANG J, SIMERT G, HANSSON JA, THYLEN U, BENGMARK S (1977) Results of a modified distal splenorenal shunt for portal hypertension. Ann Surg 185: 224
86. VAN VROONHOVEN TJ, MOLENAAR JC (1979) Distal splenorenal shunt for decompression of portal hypertension in children with cystic fibrosis. Surg Gynecol Obstet 149: 559
87. WARREN WD (1978) Ascites and portasystemic shunts (Editorial). Am J Surg 135: 607
88. WARREN WD, FOMON JJ, VIAMONTE M, ZEPPA R (1967) Preoperative assessment of portal hypertension. Ann Surg 165: 999
89. WARREN WD, ZEPPA R, FOMON JJ (1967) Selective transsplenic decompression of gastroesophageal varices by distal splenorenal shunt. Ann Surg 166: 437
90. WARREN WD, SALAM AA, FARALDO A, HUTSON D, SMITH RB (1972) End renal vein-to-splenic vein shunts for total or selective portal decompression. Surgery 72: 995
91. WARREN WD, SALAM AA, HUTSON D, ZEPPA R (1974) Selective distal splenorenal shunt, technique and results of operation. Arch Surg 108: 306
92. WESTABY S, WILKINSON SP, WARREN R, WILLIAMS R (1978) Spleen size and portal hypertension in cirrhosis. Digestion 17: 63
93. WIDRICH WC, ROBBINS AH, NABSETH DC, O'HARA ET, JOHNSON WC, LOUGHLIN KV (1976) Portal hypertension changes following selective splenorenal shunt surgery. Radiology 121: 295

94. WIDRICH WC, ROBBINS AH, JOHNSON WC, NABSETH DC (1980) Long-term follow-up of distal splenorenal shunts. Radiology 134: 341
95. ZEPPA R (1972) New surgical approaches to portal hypertension. Prog Liver Dis 4: 289
96. ZEPPA R, HUTSON DG, BERGSTRESSER PR, LEVI JU, SCHIFF ER, FINK P (1977) Survival after distal splenorenal shunt. Surg Gynecol Obstet 145: 12
97. ZEPPA R, HENSLEY GT, LEVI JU, BERGSTRESSER PR, HUTSON DG, LIVINGSTONE AS, SCHIFF ER, FINK P (1978) The comparative survival of alcoholics versus nonalcoholics after distal splenorenal shunt. Ann Surg 187: 510

# 11. Subject Index